The Secret Life of Hormones

The Secret Life of Hormones

Finding Hormone Balance for a Better Life

Dr. Zoe Zawalick

ISBN-13: 9798663250177

Dedication and Acknowledgments

Thank you, to all the women who invited me to join them on their path of healing. Thank you for sharing your stories so we can all learn and heal together.

~ Dr Zoe

To Libby Acquafresca, designer and illustrator, thank you for bringing my ideas into imagery. Thank you for taking the time to understand what I wanted to express and creating the book illustrations and cover design.

To Gina Cindaro of Cindici Photography, thank you for bringing the book cover to life with your photography!

Contents

Introduction ~ Amazing Women

Every day I see women in my medical practice who want help with low energy, sleep problems, and mood swings. They feel overwhelmed and confused by new symptoms of hot flashes, foggy brains, and an inability to handle daily stresses they had successfully managed before. They are journeying through the complex and challenging stage of perimenopause, and they want help!

Women in their 40's and 50's often have very full lives with their role of being the hub of the family as well as their many responsibilities outside of the home with work, community involvement, and caring for others. They often feel they cannot afford to have downtime or be less than their best. People are counting on them, and they need to show up. They also want to enjoy the fullness and flow of their lives and feel joy again instead of feeling exhausted, overwhelmed, and flushed.

Perimenopause is the transition stage leading up to the rite of passage that is menopause. It is the next developmental stage in a woman's life after the reproductive years. Just as puberty and adolescence brought about new challenges and pregnancy and the fertile years brought theirs, perimenopause brings both new challenges and new discoveries. Our hormones create the physiological shift to push us to evolve and grow in body, mind, and spirit. Though hormone imbalance causes much discomfort and unwanted symptoms, it also pushes us to birth the next stage of our lives.

As a doctor specializing in women's health and hormones, I want to help you understand what you are going through as your hormones change in perimenopause and how they continue to change until menopause. Let's work together to stop your suffering and help you regain peace to get back to enjoying an active and vital life. I want you to feel happy within and be able to engage with your family and friends from that place of happiness and peace instead of the irritability, anger, and anxiety that are so often a part of perimenopause.

Have you yourself had any of these experiences?

- Feeling consumed and controlled by your emotions and not knowing where they come from or what to do with them
- Feeling like you're riding the hormone rollercoaster each month and wanting it to stop
- Not being able to stay focused on your goals or intentions
- Being so tired you can't imagine having the energy to do something new or different even though you know you need to break out of the rut
- Sensing changes in your body but not knowing what to do about them - mood changes, sleep problems, new PMS symptoms and an inability to handle family or work demands that you juggled successfully before

Women come to see me in my practice when they are worn out, scared, and frustrated, and they worry they are missing all the good parts of their lives. They feel terrible on the inside and cannot enjoy all the good that is right there in front of them. They often know they need to make changes and adjustments, but they lack the energy, stamina, and focus to forge ahead and act. They need help understanding what is happening to them and what they can do about it.

I have put together this guidebook to help you get back to living and enjoying the life you have; or if your life is not what you want it to be, to regain your energy and inspiration to create the life you desire. This guidebook will help you understand what you are going through and then together we will create a realistic plan to help you reach your dreams.

We will work together to help you:

- be happy and feel good again
- feel comfortable and at home in your body maybe for the first time in your life
- have the energy and vitality to show up and be present for your life each day
- incorporate a lifestyle that supports and nourishes your beautiful body, mind, and soul
- feel inspired to take the next steps in life to feel alive and passionate

Making It Your Own – *The Practices*

I have written this book to help you understand what is going on within your body and how it influences your entire being. I have included tools to help you personalize the information and develop a wellness plan for feeling good again. Knowledge is power and having a perspective on what is happening to you is crucial to being able to change it. In addition to the information I present, I have included practices for you to internalize the information and see how this process shows up for you in your life. Then with clarity you can begin to make the adjustments needed to feel like you again. You can just read this book and end up smarter and more informed for it. But if your desire is to really see changes in your life, set aside a little time to do the practices and make this process your own. You can take time to do the practices as you go through the book or come back and do them after you have read the book all the way through. Do what works for you and make it your own. It is your journey and you get to choose the destination!

Inspiring Women, Wise Women

I have sat in many women's circles with many women – American women, English women, Gaelic women, Latinas, Native American women, European women, Jewish women, Catholic women, Christian women, Buddhist women, gay women, old women, young women, teens. I have listened to many women's stories and heard much wisdom. I have been lucky to know many aunties and grandmothers, many sisters and daughters. I have known many wise women.

I am not sure when it started, but women amaze me. The stories I have heard - of women losing babies, those yet to be born, and those with many years under their feet; partners and husbands and lovers with addiction, anger, confusion, unable to communicate their hearts; women with chronic pain, cancer, crippling anxiety, depression and many nights of lost sleep; losing their mothers, their fathers, their in-law's after years of nursing them. Women just keep going, and they keep figuring out how to live.

I see women who had so little build so much over years of dedication to a goal. They raise their children; they write beautiful songs and poetry; they raise horses and cattle and vegetables. They decorate gorgeous homes and feed families and help the kids get their homework done. They help their children find care facilities to recover from addiction, eating disorders, and mental illness.

I have worked with women to get their blood pressure under control, find a way to sleep again, stop hot flashes and night sweats and embarrassing beet red faces. We have worked to calm down the side effects of chemotherapy, radiation, and lost breasts. We discuss anxiety, depression, and years of chronically high stress. We talk of body image, weight issues, and fast food. I explain to women the symphony of their hormones – the thyroid gland, adrenal glands, ovaries and pituitary – how they work together and intersect and how their weight will not change until their hormones are in harmony.

I have assisted women in being able to become pregnant, make it through yet another miscarriage, figure out the frustrations of contraception, yeast infections and declining libido. I have assisted many women in delivering babies and being present in that holy moment when a being enters the world.

I love working with women; they impress me. They inspire me, make me laugh, and often bring tears to my eyes.

This book is my acknowledgment of all the amazing women in the world and that includes You!

Hormones Influence Our Lives

We are always becoming. From the moment we are born until the moment we breathe our last breath we are constantly becoming the next iteration of who we are. In Spanish 'becoming' is expressed as 'llegar a ser' or 'arriving to be' - we are arriving at the next destination point of who we are, who we will be next. The cycles of life move us through constant change where we are challenged to develop ourselves, learn new skills, and become adept at managing the events of life.

Whether we realize it or not, our hormones are part of this constant change, and they influence our behavior and how we see the world. Women go through many cycles of hormonal change from puberty to menopause. Each developmental and hormone cycle has its own characteristics and learning how our hormones influence us gives us the impetus we need to gracefully navigate the changing tides of life.

A Girl's First Hormonal Rite of Passage – Puberty

As women we are challenged to surf the waves of our hormones month in and month out and year in and year out. These dynamic hormones affect our emotions, thoughts, and behavior. Our hormonal journey really swings into gear in adolescence as puberty hits and overwhelms us with new emotions and sensations. Ask any pubescent girl if she is aware of the hormonal waves that pass through her and she will look at you quizzically and tell you her hormones do not affect her at all.

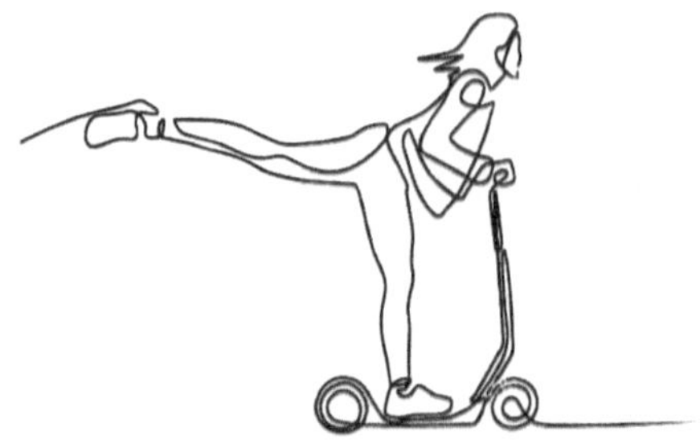

She is immersed in her hormonal experience and cannot see herself separately from her hormones. Her mother and family see the change in her, but she cannot differentiate the feelings she has and the experience of her inner world from the flood of hormones that surge through her each month.

During this time in a girl's life, she is experiencing an increase in estrogen and progesterone each month as she develops her monthly menstrual cycles. Her hormones are gearing up to prepare for fertility, but it can take months or even years for a girl's cycle to become regular and to allow for monthly ovulation when an egg is released and prepared for fertilization.

The increase in hormones during this time and their cycling each month cause increased oiliness in the skin, acne, increased belly fat and fat deposition through the hips and thighs. Girls feel the ups and downs of both estrogen and progesterone that can cause fluid retention, increased breast developmental, pelvic cramps and fullness and mood changes. We cannot separate the brain changes related to a girl developing into a teen from her progression into having menstrual cycles. They go together hand in hand.

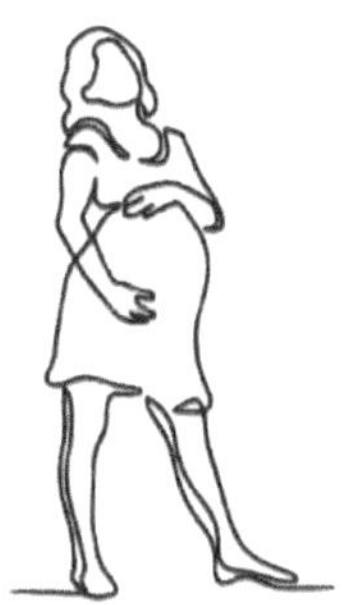

A Woman's Second Hormonal Rite of Passage – Conception and Pregnancy

The next big hormonal shift occurs when women conceive and begin pregnancy. The huge surge of hormones that build in pregnancy are much more dramatic than the hormone swings of her monthly menstrual cycles. The first trimester of pregnancy takes a woman to dramatically higher hormone levels than she has ever experienced before as the baby and placenta begin their development. Each trimester will bring significant changes in her hormones influencing her body and mind as the mother-to-be grows her baby and prepares for motherhood. Pregnancy ends in the dramatic hormone cascade of labor that allows her baby to be born followed by a great decline in hormones after labor. The baby blues and postpartum depression experienced by so many women is a testament to how these dramatic hormone swings affect the brain and mood. Hormone shifts continue in the post-partum period preparing for lactation and the eventual return of the monthly menstrual cycles.

The increased estrogen in pregnancy will initiate the bonding response in the pregnant woman helping her develop into a competent mother. The ability to put aside her own needs to care for a baby who will be dependent upon her is mediated by the hormone shifts she experiences in pregnancy. The great increase in her hormones allows for the growth and development of the baby in her womb as well as her own development into motherhood. Increased progesterone and oxytocin allow for the still mysterious initiation of labor and then later the production of breast milk as well as the development of mothering behaviors that drive a mother to care for her new child.

When you take a step back and look at a woman's hormonal life, it is quite impressive! Girls and women learn to adjust to dramatic hormone fluctuations throughout their lives. For women who experience irregular menstrual cycles, ovarian cysts, uterine fibroids and endometriosis, the challenges are even greater.

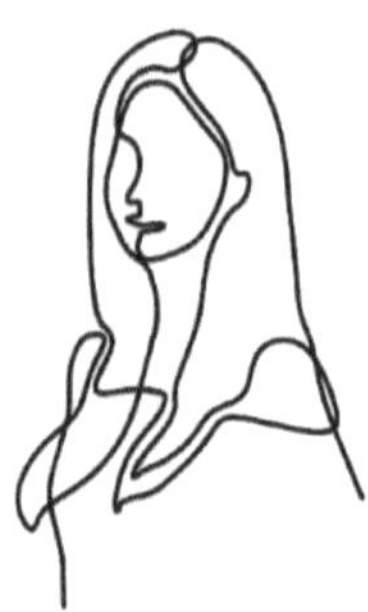

The Journey to the Third Hormonal Rite of Passage – Perimenopause

It can take women years to realize how their hormones affect their behavior from the mood swings of PMS to peri-menopausal anxiety and menopausal depression. Often women in their 40's and 50's are unaware that their hormones are responsible for their increased worry, anxiety, depression and sleep problems. They suspect that hot flashes, vaginal dryness, and a declining sex drive are caused by hormones. But the changes in their brains and moods are often misunderstood. We will delve into the intricate details of perimenopause - what it is, how it happens, how women feel during it, and how to deal with it - throughout the rest of the book.

I love helping women understand how their hormones affect their brains and thus their emotions and behavior. Research in sociology shows us that women often take sole responsibility for problems in their lives. Women can blame themselves instead of considering all the other factors that contribute to social or relational problems. This behavior of taking responsibility and assigning blame to ourselves is also hormonally directed! The female hormones estrogen and oxytocin tune up these responses in the female body to make us great moms, caretakers, and leaders of the family. Our nature through our reproductive years is to find harmony and to create a home situation where all can be cared for and nourished. Part of the change that women go through when they transition from being fertile to stopping their menstrual cycles is a decline in estrogen and oxytocin that changes their nurturing behavior.

When women understand that the changes in their emotions and behavior are strongly influenced by hormones, they breathe a sigh of relief. Secretly they thought they were crazy. They thought they were losing it, and they would be lost forever. They can finally exhale when they understand that this is just a transition phase mediated by their hormones and part of the journey of womanhood.

In perimenopause a woman may feel like she is no longer in control of her behavior and her hormones are shaking her reality. As her hormone levels decline, the longings and passions she felt earlier in life change, and she may start to feel depressed or bored. She can feel like the best part of life has passed her by; her importance and enthusiasm have diminished, and she cannot imagine what could possibly be next that would make her happy again. But the story does not end here!

She is still becoming! In this very moment, a new part of her is being gestated. She is pregnant with who she will become. The latest update is about to be released! Take a moment to remember how uncomfortable pregnancy was or if you have not birthed babies, how uncomfortable you were when your period started for the first time. As thrilling as it was, it was also terrifying, disconcerting, and strange. This current pregnancy and subsequent delivery of your new self will also be uncomfortable and scary at times. You may not know if you can get through it, and you assuredly do not know HOW you will get through it. But that is why you are reading this book – to learn HOW you will birth your new self and create the life you so badly desire!

The times in a woman's life when she is shifting from one hormonal stage to another can feel daunting. She experiences new sensations and feelings and must learn new coping mechanisms to adjust to her new reality. Often women are unaware of what they are going through internally with their hormones, they just feel bad and blame themselves. We are constantly adjusting and learning new strategies to cope with our ever-changing internal environment, not to mention our external environments!

Our Inner and Outer Worlds

We have both an interior world and an exterior world. Our lives go through phases of development, learning, and challenges both externally in the events of our lives and internally in our bodies. These two elements are not separate. In fact, our inner world and our outer world affect one another. Our external lives mirror what is going on in our bodies, and our bodies help evolve and shape our external lives.

When we look at children it is so clear how rapidly they develop and go through stages. They are teething, learning to sit up, eat, crawl and then eventually walk. We then mark their development with the passage of each school year and next grade level achieved. In late childhood or adolescence, puberty marks dramatic change and then through adolescence and early adulthood the more subtle changes of development include gaining independence, moving away from home, completing advanced studies in work or education.

In Western culture we stop measuring growth and development once adulthood has been reached. So how do we measure our progression when we have finished our education; our children have grown up; we have mastered our work; and our relationships are well established? We do not realize that we are still developing. Now the growth is internal, underneath the surface and more difficult to perceive. Instead of forward movement we may feel like we are slowly falling apart: wrinkles are showing up, hairs are turning gray, vision is less acute, and energy has decreased. It is one thing to progress and advance in growth but to digress and slide backward is quite another! How do we understand the positive aspects of what is changing within us and not focus solely on what is falling away?

Many women feel betrayed by their bodies during perimenopause not realizing that their bodies are trying to help them develop new ways of being. As our hormones slow down and decrease in their production, we are meant to find a new pace, a new rhythm for the next part of life. If we befriend the body and see it is our ally, we can work with it and create a new place of balance. Having an attitude of curiosity about what the body is trying to tell us instead of being critical about how the body is changing will allow us to change more gracefully. There is much to be gained from changing our daily habits, but sometimes we are afraid to let go of how it has been. We do not know what it will look like to do things differently and that can feel scary.

Our changing hormones are meant to shift our focus from the external world back into our internal world. They ask of us to stop looking outside of ourselves and stop spending our energy worrying about and caring for others. Now is the time to come back home to ourselves, to care for our internal world.

My goal is to help you understand how your hormones influence you and how you can balance and support your hormonal health to make you happy again as you navigate the twists and turns of life. It takes a lot of courage, stamina, and determination to live life and keep going amidst the turbulence of the outer world and the disruptive hormonal changes within our bodies. I want you to understand and a greater perspective on what is happening inside your body and use it to your advantage instead of suffering through it. Then you will have tools to help you navigate the rough terrain of perimenopause and find joy and peace once again.

Rebecca's Story

Rebecca's story is one I see frequently of how the changing hormones of perimenopause affect the quality and experience of everyday life. Rebecca came into my practice appearing anxious and uptight. She was married, owned her own part-time business teaching music classes, was raising her two daughters and felt she had a good life. But regardless of how good life was on the outside, Rebecca could not shake the sense that something was terribly wrong on the inside. She woke at night in a full panic – sweating and with her heart racing for no apparent reason. It would take her hours to fall back asleep going around and around in her mind not knowing how she would be able to meet the challenges of the next day. She had had to give up teaching classes because of her fatigue and foggy brain. She constantly worried about her family and was becoming impatient with her daughters. She felt guilty for being negative and irritable with her family, and they were frustrated with her, but she could not change her behavior no matter how hard she tried. She felt out of control, exhausted, and fearful about her health and mental state.

I assessed Rebecca's hormones and discovered where the hormone imbalance was. She was in the middle of perimenopause and was ramping up to the next level of progesterone decline. We started her on natural supplements to assist her endocrine system as well as adding a small amount of bioidentical progesterone cream. I did not see Rebecca again until a year later and was surprised to see her come into the office with a huge smile on her face. She appeared relaxed, in control, and balanced. She thanked me and told me how the adjustments we had made in her hormones brought her life back. She was able to teach classes again; she slept well; her patience and sense of ease were back and so was the knowledge that life was good. She did not need much to maintain her health and hormone balance at this point. She had just needed some fine tuning to bring her changing hormones back into balance.

Practice 1 – Telling Your Story

With this first practice start a journal, notebook, or new folder on your computer to store all your Practices in one place.

Find a few minutes of calm to allow yourself to get quiet inside. Take a few slow, deep breathes then begin.

What is your story as you went through the Rites of Passage of Puberty and Menarche and then later Fertility and Pregnancy?

Puberty and Your First Period

Think back to puberty. Do you remember when you first heard about girls having their periods?

How did you feel when you were anticipating the start of your period? Was it scary? Exciting? Horrifying?

What were those first years of your period like for you? Did you take it in stride or did it have a big impact on your life? Did your period come every month or was it sporadic?

Did you start before your friends or after your friends? Did you feel different about yourself and about the world once you had started your period?

Fertility and Pregnancy

What are your first memories around being able to get pregnant? Did you cherish the idea of becoming a mother or did the idea having a child make you uncomfortable? Was becoming a mother a major desire for you in your life or did you want to put your time and energy into other endeavors?

How did you feel about getting pregnant? Were you able to get pregnant easily or did you need assistance? Was it stressful? Exciting? Scary? Joyful? If you had multiple children, what did the process of pregnancy and birthing children mean to you? As you went through this enormous life change of birthing children, how did your thoughts and feelings about yourself change? Did you think of the world differently?

If you were unable to become pregnant but wanted to get pregnant, how did you feel about not being able to get pregnant? How did you feel about yourself and the world when you were not able to become pregnant?

If you did not go through pregnancy and did not want to become pregnant, what was it like seeing friends and family go through pregnancy? Did your feelings about yourself and the world change as you went through this time in your life?

What are Perimenopause and Menopause?

What is perimenopause? There are not many words that cause more confusion and disconnect than perimenopause. Think of perimenopause as being analogous to puberty but in reverse. Puberty is when the hormones ramp up, and we become fertile and start our periods. Perimenopause is the opposite of puberty; it is the ending of our menstrual cycles and fertility. Just as it was confusing and disorienting to go through puberty so it is as we go through perimenopause.

Perimenopause refers to the time frame when our bodies are shifting from high hormone levels that allow us to be fertile and have periods to lower hormone levels that cause our periods to stop. The body needs to make this shift because if we were to remain fertile forever, we would not be able to live as long. As we become older, the body shifts its priorities. It moves from baby making ability to maintaining the heart, bones, and brain for longer life.

Perimenopause begins in the mid to late thirties for some women and by the early forties for most women. The entire process of perimenopause can last from 5 to 15 years! This is a process and transition not an overnight shift. Some women will stop having periods in their forties while others continue having periods into their mid to late-50's.

It is this variability in the timing and presentation of perimenopause that causes so much confusion. Many women do not realize they are going through perimenopause when they are. That is fine if they are feeling relatively good and balanced. But if they are starting to feel crazy, sleep deprived and confused about what is happening in their bodies, it is worthwhile to learn about the process of perimenopause. When we understand what our bodies are going through, we have more compassion for ourselves and can start to see ourselves from a larger perspective.

What does perimenopause look like?

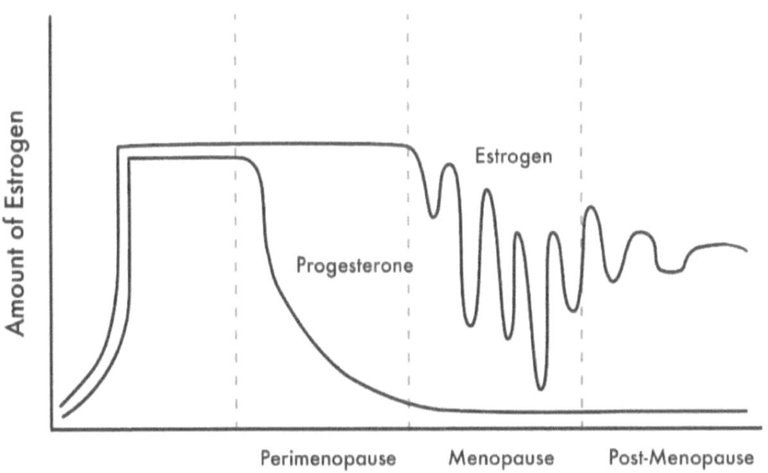

The graph above is a good representation perimenopause. See the squiggly line? That is your estrogen during perimenopause! The dramatic changes in estrogen from month to month take you up some steep climbs and terrifying plunges. No wonder you feel crazy at times! (Later in this chapter I will describe how estrogen affects you).

Perimenopause is like this: you are cruising along in your life busy with raising kids, being in a primary relationship or doing it on your own, working/volunteering/creating and suddenly it is just too hard. You stop sleeping or wake up throughout the night without being able to fall back asleep. You are grouchy or touchy and this time you really do not know why. Nothing has changed in your life, but you feel different. You are frustrated and irritated by your family members, work stress is just too much, you feel a little out of control and know it is not because of something on the outside. It is about something inside of you, and you are not sure what it is. You do not like it, and you also do not know what to do about it.

For many women perimenopause causes increased irritability or even anxiety; trouble sleeping; an increase in the amount or severity of PMS symptoms. It does not usually hit hard right away. Instead it creeps up on you and slowly influences your life often in ways you do not expect and do not necessarily like. But the good news is – there is a lot you can do to help yourself, and you are doing one of them right now! Learning about yourself and what your body is going through is the first step to making sense of this process and finding your way back to happiness and calm.

What is menopause?

Menopause means the cessation of periods. We consider a woman to be in menopause once she has not had a period for 13 consecutive months. Many women will go 6 months or more without a period during perimenopause and then have a period out of the blue. She will not be in menopause until she has gone more than a year with no periods. Post-menopausal means the same thing as menopause - a woman has passed the 13-month mark without having a period. At this point the hormones have reached a stable point (and an all-time low) where a woman is beyond the hormone rollercoaster of perimenopause.

15

Hormones as Catalysts for Transformation

Hormones act as catalysts for change. They influence our physical bodies, emotions, and behavior to help us evolve through each stage of our lives. With each rite of passage from puberty, fertility, perimenopause and on into menopause, our hormones prepare us for transformation. We blossom from a family oriented girl in childhood to becoming a teen with a different world view in adolescence and then into fertility and the creation of our own homes and families. Becoming a mother is an incredible transformation where we allow ourselves to expand physically as well as spiritually both for ourselves and for this new child entering the world. We put aside our individual personality to make space for new life. The process of pregnancy makes us small; as our bellies grow large, our individual ego moves to the background.

When our hormones shift in perimenopause, our emotions and behavior also shift. It is time to change our focus. From the outward focus on children, spouses, and family we now need to move that focus back to ourselves to attend to our personal wants and needs. We need that attention and care to rebuild ourselves to prepare for the next stages in our life. We enter this new phase with all the life experiences that mothering and caring for relationships has given us. We are more balanced having experienced both the personal self as well as the collective self who cares for others. Now we can merge these two experiences - Self and Mother - and evolve to the next stage of womanhood with an expanded perspective.

Understanding the Endocrine System

Our hormones are made and released by glands in the body called endocrine glands. The ovaries, pituitary, adrenals, thyroid and pancreas are all endocrine glands that produce and secrete hormones. These glands communicate with each other and send signals to one another to increase production of some hormones while decreasing others. The brain organizes and transmits many of these messages but the glands themselves can also send messages to one another and to the brain.

I like to compare the endocrine system to an orchestra with the brain as conductor and each gland an individual instrument needed for the orchestra to play complex and beautiful music. Just as the conductor will motion for the saxophones to start playing when the flutes stop playing – more percussion, less strings, then more wood winds, less horns – the brain will sense when a hormone such as cortisol is high and in response will send a message to the ovaries to lower progesterone levels thereby affecting estrogen release delaying ovulation. The endocrine system is an interactive and ever-changing piece of music producing inspiring pieces when all the instruments are in tune and unpleasant, irritating sounds when the instruments are out of sync with one another.

It is this complex interaction between the glands and their hormones that wreak such havoc in perimenopause. We need to keep in mind these complex interactions in the endocrine system to be able to bring all the hormones back into balance.

The Endocrine Glands

Ovaries – Women have two ovaries, one on each side of the pelvis that take turns secreting an egg each month during our fertile years. These little almond shaped glands are responsible for many of the hormonal ups and downs we face each month throughout our menstrual cycling. The ovaries produce and secrete the sex hormones estrogen, progesterone, and testosterone. Many women develop cysts in the ovaries at some point in their lives which negatively impacts the production of progesterone causing more intense PMS, fertility issues, and problems in perimenopause.

Adrenal glands – the adrenal glands which look like little mushrooms located on top of the kidneys are crucial for the functioning of the body. The adrenals produce cortisol, aldosterone, epinephrine, norepinephrine and the androgens: precursors to estrogen and testosterone. The adrenal hormones help us deal with stress – from physical pain and disease to mental/emotional stress. The adrenal glands are also affected by stress and our daily habits of caffeine consumption, inadequate rest, and chronic anxiety.

Not only are the adrenal hormones important for our day to day function during our reproductive years but in menopause, the adrenals also take over hormone production from the ovaries. The adrenals will never make the same amount of sex hormones made by the ovaries, but their small production becomes significant in menopause.

Thyroid gland – The thyroid is located in the front of the neck and works in conjunction with the adrenals to support our whole-body energy. Thyroid hormones regulate our metabolism and cellular function affecting fat burning, cellular repair, cholesterol metabolism and serum calcium balance. The thyroid is often thrown off balance by major changes in sex hormone such as puberty, pregnancy, labor and perimenopause. At these hormonally challenging times, an imbalance in thyroid hormones can cause weight gain, hair loss and low energy.

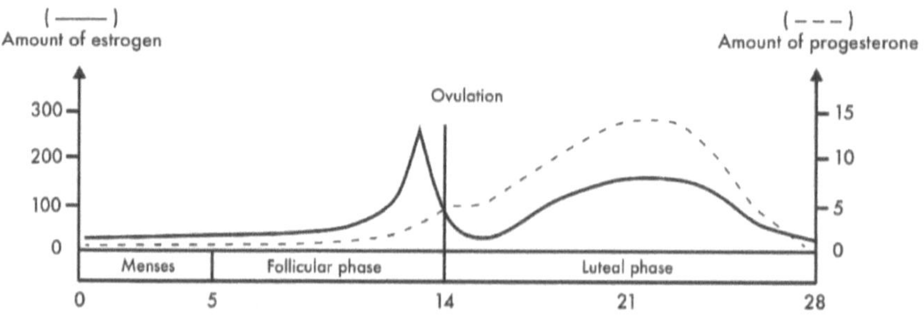

Women's Sex Hormones

Estrogen – Estrogen is the lay term we use to refer to the whole family of estrogens, the feminizing hormone found in both women and men. The strongest and most discussed estrogen is estradiol. When we test hormone levels with either a blood test or saliva test, we always check estradiol levels since it has the most potent effect in the body and is the most studied of all the female estrogens. Estriol and estrone are two other estrogens you may hear about. Research on estriol demonstrates its protective effects on the body as well as its safety for use in women who have had breast cancer. Estrone is an estrogen that has more potential for having negative effects in the body, so we want to keep estrone levels low.

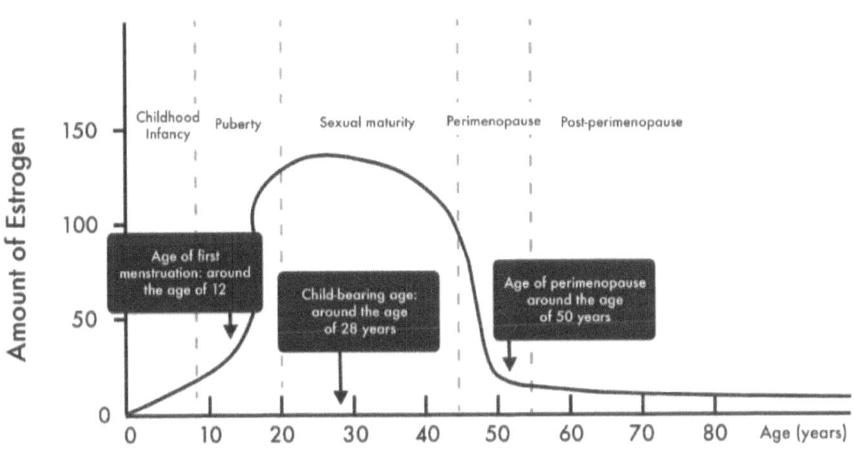

What estrogen does in the body:

Supports elasticity of skin, vagina, and joints

Moisturizes and hydrates tissue including skin and eyes

Maintains bladder tone

Supports a normal sleep cycle

Gives us a feeling of emotional well being

Thickens the endometrium, the lining of the uterus which is shed during menstruation

Supports hair growth

Supports neurotransmitter production for memory and cognitive

function
Supports bone density

Progesterone – though not as widely talked about as estrogen, progesterone has major actions in our body. Progesterone is a major player in ovulation, when the egg is released each month to allow for fertilization and conception. After the egg is released, the leftover follicle that released the egg starts to make progesterone. Women with ovarian cysts or who have problems ovulating, do not make sufficient progesterone and have more problems with irregular menstrual cycles, fertility, and more intense PMS symptoms including breast tenderness, cramping, and headaches.

Progesterone is the first hormone to change dramatically in perimenopause. Women often think their symptoms are due to estrogen changes, but it is actually a decline in progesterone production that causes many of the early symptoms in perimenopause. As progesterone production declines or becomes more erratic women experience hot flashes or night sweats making it more difficult to stay asleep during the night. Low progesterone makes a woman feel more irritable, more anxious, and less patient.

What progesterone does in the body:
Acts as an anti-inflammatory
Helps build bone density
Calms the brain by decreasing anxiety
Supports normal sleep cycles
Regulates the menstrual cycle
Maintains fluid balance and water retention in the body
Supports orgasms

Testosterone – women have much lower levels of testosterone than men but even at low levels, testosterone exerts a powerful influence. A small amount of testosterone goes a long way in keeping our bones and tissues strong; maintaining muscle mass; and supporting energy and stamina. Testosterone levels vary greatly from woman to woman. Some women with higher lifelong testosterone levels will look younger, have less emotional lability, tend toward higher amounts of facial and body hair, acne and higher blood pressure. Women with testosterone on the lower end of the spectrum will have more mood swings, more flexibility and less muscle and bone strength. They may tend toward lower libidos and more gentle dispositions.

What testosterone does in the body:
Strengthens bladder, labia, and vaginal tissue
Supports the libido or sex drive
Strengthens muscles and helps maintain muscle density
Provides physical endurance
Maintains bone density

Symptoms of Hormones Gone Awry

Hormones interact with one another in an intricate and complex fashion. When all hormones are being produced and secreted normally, the glands communicate amicably and support one another in maintaining hormonal balance and well-being. The brain receives the feedback message that 'all is well'. But when one hormone becomes imbalanced it affects all the other hormones downstream, and the brain gets the message that there is a problem. The brain (particularly the pituitary and hypothalamus) will then send out signals to the glands to fix the problem. Here are some of the symptoms associated with imbalances (either too much or too little) of specific hormones.

When estrogen is out of balance, it can cause:
Weight gain that is difficult to lose
Depression and mood swings
Sleep problems
Poor memory, foggy brain, and problems thinking clearly

Hair loss
Dry skin, increased wrinkles
Vaginal dryness
Pain with sex
Bladder infections

When progesterone is out of balance, it can cause:
Anxiety, worry
Heart palpitations
Problems sleeping
Hot flashes and night sweats
Panic attacks
Water retention
Breast tenderness
Difficulty having an orgasm

When testosterone is out of balance, it can cause:
Weakness
Poor physical stamina
Low libido
Incontinence
Weight gain around middle
Acne
Increased facial hair growth

Adrenal symptoms:
Lightheaded or dizzy
Low blood sugar
Low blood pressure
Fatigue
Difficulty waking in morning
Nervousness, anxiety
A sense of being wired and tired

Feeling stressed, overreacting to stress, inability to cope with stress

Thyroid symptoms:
Hair loss or thinning
Dry skin
Fatigue, tiredness
Depression
Cold body temperature
Loss of outer 1/3 of eyebrows
Constipation

Assessing Hormone Status

As you can see, hormone balance is crucial to health and wellness. I recommend working with a practitioner who can assess your hormone status and provide you with treatment to bring your hormones back into balance. Practitioners vary widely in their experience and expertise in endocrine function. Choose a practitioner who is up to date and well versed in endocrine issues. Ask what kind of lab work they use to assess hormones and how they treat endocrine issues. The most experienced practitioners will use blood tests, salivary tests, or urine tests to measure hormones.

Your doctor will assess your symptoms and look for patterns of symptoms that signal a dysfunction in one of more of the endocrine glands. Then they will order specific lab tests that measure hormone levels to clarify where the imbalance is. Once the diagnosis is made, treatment can focus on returning the endocrine system to full function and alleviating your symptoms. In my practice I commonly test for the following hormones when I am assessing a woman's endocrine function:

Estradiol
Estrone
Progesterone

Testosterone
DHEA
Cortisol
Thyroid stimulating hormone
Free T3
Free T4

Hitting Menopause Hard – *My Story*

I have worked with thousands of women and heard their stories of how life, health issues, and hormones have rocked their worlds. I have worked with women through pregnancy and labor and have also seen how they traversed these intense and life changing events. But it was not until I went through pregnancy and delivered my own son that I knew in my body what it was like to be pregnant and give birth. There is one level of knowing that academics and practice can teach us and another level that can only be reached through personal experience.

I was very familiar with the changes that women went through in perimenopause through my medical education and many years of practice. I, myself, started hot flashes and had a drop in progesterone early on in perimenopause so I could personally relate to what many of my patients were experiencing. But the estrogen crash that occurred when I went through menopause hit me harder than I expected. I could see my estrogen was diminishing over time but when it bottomed out completely, it took me with it! Even with my awareness of the life changes I was going through at the time: turning 50, my only son graduating from high school, and completing 20 years of medical practice – I was still surprised by what it felt like for my estrogen to hit rock bottom. It felt like all the life had gone out of me. Nothing excited me anymore. Everything felt blah and gray there was nothing I could think of to get excited about. This was different from situational depression, it was more like watching a movie where all the color had been drained out. I could see this and understand it intellectually, but I could not change it. I really wondered what life would be like if it carried on this way. It just did not feel very inspiring or meaningful anymore.

Every woman has her own experience during perimenopause and into menopause. Some women go through irritability and terrible sleep problems that leave them with short fuses especially for their children and partners. Other women get angry and start to eat away at their personal relationships or co-workers as they battle the urge to tell everyone off. Some women step into mental emotional instability and begin to understand how their mothers, aunts, or grandmas went a little crazy (or went into full-fledged mental illness) in their menopausal years. Many women lose their sex drive – some care and some do not. But every woman changes. A woman takes what life gives her including a changing body and a changing mind and she creates the next step. Often this is not done calmly or gracefully but with tears and sweat and an inner stamina that only comes from years of living life and climbing mountains and figuring out how to keep going even when it's not fun anymore.

If you are going through any or all of this, know that you are not alone. You are a woman walking the heroine's path. You may not look like the magazine or social media image of the perfect woman but you are the woman who continues to walk through life, discover herself, and become the next iteration of who she is. You get to define what you are birthing - your creation, your art, your beauty.

Practice 2 – The Perimenopausal Years

What is your experience with perimenopause: are you experiencing hormonal change yourself? Have you seen it in your friends, sisters, mother or aunts? What have you learned from other women who are going through this change or have already been through it?

If you are seeing hormonal changes within yourself, describe what is different? Is your period changing or have PMS symptoms changed? Are you experiencing hot flashes, unaccounted for irritability, or sleep problems?

As you read over the symptoms associated with estrogen and progesterone and their actions in the body, do you see any patterns with your own symptoms?

If you have been through perimenopause and are now in menopause, think back about what your transition was like. Did you know what you were going through at the time? What was it like going through the body and mind changes? How did you think and feel about yourself as you went through these changes? For many women, this transition takes many years. As you look back can you see your progression through perimenopause and how you changed during that time? Do you feel differently about your world now that you are in menopause?

Practice 3 – Tracking Symptoms

Start a symptom journal or load a health app onto your phone where you can keep track of symptoms. You do not need to know why you are having symptoms or if any of your discomforts are related to hormonal change. Just keep a list of problems that bother you on a consistent basis that you can share with your health practitioner.

If you are still having a period either monthly or irregularly, download an app to track your periods. Many apps also help you track other symptoms throughout the month.

Keep notes about changes in sleep, new headaches patterns, herpes outbreaks, yeast infections and mood changes.

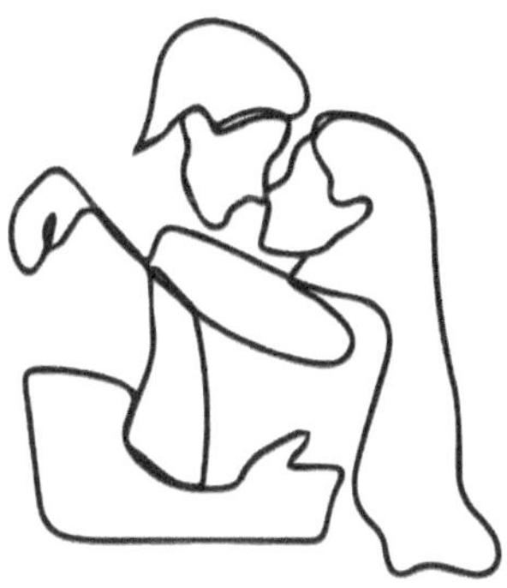

The Hot Topics ~ Sex, Aging, and Andropause

Sex and Libido The drive to engage sexually is part mystery and part physiology, part cultural conditioning and part individual experience. Our sex drive or libido is a complex, multi-faceted drive. As a doctor I look at all the elements that make up the sex drive and sexual response – hormone levels and health issues, emotional needs and relationship issues as well as the spiritual drives to connect and explore a deeper experience together. All of these components influence our sexual desire and behavior from our youth through the post-menopausal years. We must consider the dynamic flow of hormones as well as the shifts in our emotional and spiritual needs to get a full perspective on how our libido and sexual expression change over our lifetimes.

As teens and young adults, we may have felt the thrill of sexual desire and the urge for sexual experiences. The hormonal surges of puberty initiate our libido - that exciting, uncontrollable, overwhelming and sometimes confusing sensation. This huge life force moves through us and affects our behavior including the newfound desire to engage with others in previously unknown ways. This inner desire drives us toward connecting physically and emotionally and engaging in relationships.

The novelty of early love and sexual encounters is eventually replaced with longer lasting relationships which shifts our desire as we establish routines or patterned sexual engagements with our mates. If sex then creates a family, we are now faced with hormonal, emotional, and lifestyle shifts which again impact our longing for physical intimacy. Our yearning for physical intimacy can be superseded by our children's needs and our connection to them again shifts our libido and connection with our mates.

The perimenopausal years coincide with children growing up and becoming more independent, and menopause comes as children are leaving home and emptying the nest. We may find ourselves alone again with our mates after many years of raising a family and parenting. Here again our physical bodies are changing at the same time our emotional and spiritual needs are changing. Maybe this is not such a coincidence after all!

Perimenopause is a dynamic time for many women's libidos. Some women will feel an increase in sexual desire while others experience a sharp decline in libido from perimenopause to menopause. One of the most common complaints I hear from women in perimenopause is of declining libidos. What they really say is, "I don't feel anything anymore; it's gone." Nothing, zilch, zero, absent. Some women feel guilty for not wanting to engage sexually when her partner does. Others feel pressure to maintain a regular sex routine to support her relationship even when she herself feels no sexual desire. Some women speak of a new distance from her partner that was previously bridged through sexual connection; others are frustrated and grieve the loss of pleasure and joy they found in the sexual experience.

For some women a decline in libido is a relief especially if they have been uncomfortable with sex, have had a history of sexual abuse, or have long standing anger or resentment toward their partner. For women whose low libidos correlate with their partner's diminished desire, new satisfaction can be found in cuddling, kissing, and holding one another. Sex is no longer needed to meet their physical, emotional, and spiritual needs.

For couples who have a mismatch in desire and cannot easily discuss sex or find ways to fulfill each other's needs, the change in regularity of sexual contact can drive a wedge into the relationship. Many men and some women feel more connected through the experience of sexual intimacy than in any other way. No matter what form intimacy takes – oral sex, intercourse, foreplay, touching or massaging each other – it leads to feelings of emotional and spiritual closeness. For some there is no replacement for sexual intimacy. It is important for each relationship to discover what their unique needs are and work together to fulfill these needs for both partners.

Instead of being intimidated by this problem and turning away from it or from one's partner, it can be very helpful to sit down and have an honest and caring conversation about sex and what your needs are and what that connection means to each of you. When one partner realizes that a decrease in libido does not mean they are loved less, it can lessen the blow. Then other avenues for expressing love can be discovered. When both partners can calmly and openly discuss what they want and need from affection or physical intimacy, there is room to find solutions. Even the act of being willing to talk about it and listen to one another builds intimacy and trust and that in and of itself can stimulate the libido and desire to connect in more intimate ways. It takes a degree of vulnerability and willingness to do something unfamiliar but attempting to do something new is exactly what is needed to build closeness, desire, and stimulate that internal fire of mystery and connection. Staying in the same routine will not reignite new sexual desire. We must be willing to stretch and to entertain novelty to bring fresh air into our bedroom, and our relationship.

Problems with Sex

As the body changes, sex also needs to change. Here are the common problems women face in menopause:

Vaginal dryness – at some point in a woman's life she will experience vaginal dryness. This can run the spectrum from mild dryness managed by vaginal lubricants to severe dryness that creates pain with intercourse. For women with severe vaginal dryness and atrophy, topical hormones, suppositories, or systemic hormones may be needed.

Some couples find oral sex to be more comfortable and satisfying than vaginal intercourse as they go through aging changes. With vaginal dryness and changes in men's erectile function, oral sex may be an avenue of more pleasure and less discomfort.

Bladder infections – Decreasing estrogen in a woman's body causes thinning of the tissue around her urethra. This allows bacteria to enter the urethra and cause bladder infections more easily. Increased dryness of tissue and thinning of tissue are both at fault here. Using water-based lubricants to decrease friction around the urethra, washing well before and after sex, and using hormones to strengthen and moisturize the labia and vaginal tissue can all help prevent bladder infections.

Orgasm – The ability to orgasm is a hormonal as well as psychological event. Lower hormones in menopause can inhibit a woman's ability to orgasm or lengthen the time it takes her to reach climax. There are many factors that play into having an orgasm: decreased circulation in the pelvic area, decreased hormones, discomfort from dryness, fear of incontinence during orgasm. If orgasm becomes difficult, a woman may also become anxious about her performance further inhibiting her ability to reach orgasm. This same situation can happen with men and erectile dysfunction.

Practice 4 – Sex

How is sex going for you? What is your history around sex: has it been more pleasurable or painful? How is it changing at this point in your life?

Has your libido changed? Do you dread sex or miss sex?

Are you having any problems with sex?

Have libido changes or problems with sex impacted your relationship with your partner? Does your partner seem to be going through any changes with sex or libido?

Consider whether it would be beneficial to engage in a conversation with your partner around sex. Would making adjustments to your love making make it more pleasurable for each of you?

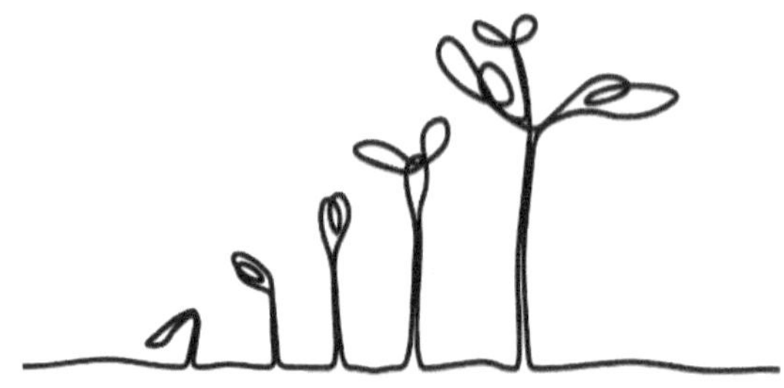

Aging – No One Wants to Get Old

When I was a new doctor and starting practice at thirty years old, I was surprised that women did not talk about menopause amongst themselves. I wanted to encourage them to share their experiences with their friends and sisters so they could support each other and normalize this hormonal life transition. I thought it would solve many problems if women could rally around one another as they moved through this rite of passage.

Fifteen years later, in my mid-forties, I again tried to bring women together in small groups to learn about perimenopause and menopause and to support each other. I had written my first book about perimenopause and was excited to provide women with tools to help them through the problems they came to talk to me about every day in my practice. What I found was that many 40 and 50 year old's did not know what perimenopause meant and it was not until women had stopped their periods that they were willing to learn about what they had already gone through! Women did not even want to utter the word menopause until they were well done with their periods and then it was only mentioned in hushed tones. I could not figure out what the disconnect was.

Now in my 50's, I understand why women are loathe to embrace the terms perimenopause and menopause. It is all about aging. Perimenopause and menopause mean that we are not young, fertile women anymore. We do not have plump, tight skin, and shiny bright complexions. Our hair is not as full and luxurious as it once was and our vaginas are becoming dry. Who wants to admit this is what she is going through? No woman does.

I started to become aware that as we age, we begin to fade. Our beauty fades, our color fades, our hair fades, our vibrancy fades, our overt sexuality fades, our powers of attraction fade, our power in the world fades and our competitiveness fades. We fade. What a tragedy this can feel like! I think it is the immensity of the issue of aging that keeps us from embracing the rite of menopause until we can deny it no longer. We do not want to prematurely age or give up on our youthfulness until we can no longer deny that we have moved past it.

Having grown up in Southern California, the epitome of image consciousness and youth worship, I realized how much pressure women were under to maintain their youthfulness to 'stay attractive'. When we are younger, we think our youthfulness and vitality will last, and we will somehow avoid aging. I was also under this spell, thinking that my commitment to health and vitality would carry me through. I never realized that I too would fade. My peers and I would be replaced by the younger generation, the new moms, the new graduates, the young, eager professionals who had so much energy and vigor and new ideas! And they knew how to use their phone app's and were active on social media and knew the new styles and lingo that were a little unfamiliar to us. What a loss this was to realize that our power would fade.

American culture is still based on the new, young, and vital. By global standards we are still a young country and we worship new ideas, innovation, change and new stimulus. We are the easiest country in the world in which to be an entrepreneur and to succeed. The pilgrims left behind tradition and dogma with their rigid structures and beliefs to create a new world, and we continue with those same values. So what do we do when we find that we are getting older, and we are no longer the innovators?

As we move through this rite of passage, our mothers and aunties pass the baton to us and encourage us to reassess, take inventory, create anew. It is time to evolve. What we have garnered up to this point is life experience. We have mastered skills and built mental fortitude. We have lived through many seasons and have a perspective born out of living life and traipsing through hardship and failures and successes and letting go of what did not work and walking forward with the knowledge of what did. This tenacity, self-knowledge, and confidence gained only through a life fully lived, give us the skills to move forward and create anew.

There are many ways to deal with aging. We can embrace it, deny it, optimize it or delay it. The anti-aging movement in medicine, a new field of medicine growing stronger and more affluent by the day speaks loudly to our discomfort with aging. The industry knows we do not want to age, and they have a wealth of products, procedures and devices to delay or seemingly avoid the whole process. I wonder if we are fortunate to have these resources or not. They provide us opportunities to redefine aging but also set up expectations to continue to look and act young while avoiding stepping into the next stage of our lives. We color our hair to keep the gray away and help us look years younger. Estheticians, dermatologists and medical spas lighten age spots, erase lines, and lift sagging skin. Collagen and super foods boost energy, ease our aches, and help us look younger on the outside even as we change and morph on the inside.

Having practiced for more than twenty years, I have seen my patients age. We see our parents, neighbors, friends, political figures, athletes, actors and musicians all age if they are fortunate to live long enough. It is sobering to see people you have known for many years grow older and adapt to a changing body and changing life. People close to us die and our parents now require our care and attention. Our peer group changes from being the top athletes and superstars to becoming the trainers and mentors to the new generation of stars and eventually becoming regular people. We step back to allow the new generation of performers and achievers, some of whom may be our children to step into the spotlight. While it is exciting to see our children and younger friends grow up and thrive, it is not so exciting or pleasurable to see our mentors, coaches, and respected figures wither and become frail. It is a process that we may come to slowly, the acceptance that life is temporary, and one day we will all meet the same fate. But as we become more comfortable with this deep understanding and eventually accept this reality, we can find freedom and even comfort in the process of aging. When we stop struggling against it and pushing it away, we can step more solidly into the flow of life. We have today and the present moment, and these alone can motivate us to create our next step.

Many of my senior patients have been role models for me and are redefining aging, not by denying it but by modeling a new way ahead. The Baby Boomer generation is more active than their parents - living longer, working longer, and being involved with their communities and families later in life. They are also increasing their level of fitness and overall health in their senior years, something we have never seen before. My senior patients have taught me about the vital importance of our minds – our mindsets, beliefs, and inner stamina – and how to keep using those skills to adapt to change within ourselves and our lives.

Though aging is not a topic we eagerly await, we must find a way to begin to work with it as we journey through perimenopause and into menopause. We have the opportunity to define what this process will mean to us. To move into the next phase of life, we must find some level of acceptance and peace to decide how we want to live it. We cannot avoid or deny it anymore, but we can decide how we want to think about it and live it.

Practice 5 – The Question of Aging

The topic of aging is a huge one. What came up for you as you read the section on aging? What feelings and thoughts arose? What was uncomfortable or downright frightening?

How have you felt about aging up to this point in your life? Consider what role models you have regarding getting older. Are there some that inspire you? What is it about them that makes you feel good? If you do not know anyone who is aging in a way that you want to emulate, consider expanding your view. Actively seek out a model of healthy aging - a neighbor, a friend's parent, a coworker, an actor, an athlete, the usher at your local performing arts center. Notice what you respect about them. As you put your intention on finding people who embody your ideals around aging, you will find them. They may show up in the most unexpected places!

Begin to describe how you want to be as you get older. How do you want to feel? What do you want to be doing? What types of activities sound interesting? What new endeavors could you put time into that you have not had time for yet? How do you want your body to feel? Will you change your style – hair, makeup, or clothing? These are questions that will take years to answer fully, but as we begin to consider positive aspects of aging, we change our relationship from one of fear and avoidance to one of acceptance and positivity.

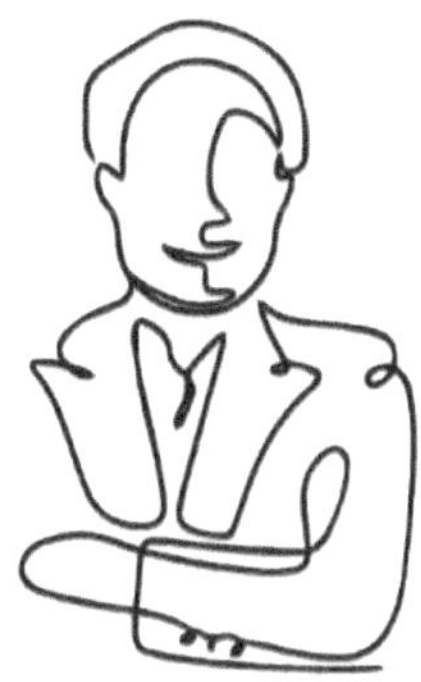

Andropause – The Male Menopause

Men go through their own version of hormonal change called andropause. Andropause refers to a decline in the production of androgens or male hormones. The most predominant androgen is testosterone, but you may have also heard of DHEA, an adrenal hormone that is also an androgen. Androgens are the hormones responsible for the masculinizing effects on the body, and they are also precursors to estrogens. Men do not completely stop producing testosterone during their lifetimes, but testosterone levels decline with age. The degree to which testosterone levels decline varies from man to man with some men experiencing huge downward spirals in testosterone production over a few short years while others have only a mild decrease in testosterone over decades. While most women will have significantly lower estrogen and progesterone levels after menopause, not all men will end up with low testosterone levels after andropause.

Men and Testosterone

To better understand testosterone's effect on men, let's look at how it changes throughout a man's life. In young boys, testosterone levels are low, but when a boy goes through puberty in late childhood or during adolescence, his testosterone will increase up to 30 times! The dramatic increase in this powerful hormone significantly changes a boy's behavior, personality, and perspective on life. He will feel more energy, an increase in power, uncontrollable erections, sexual thoughts and urges. Testosterone's effect on his body will increase perspiration, hair growth, oil secretions in the skin and acne while also affecting blood sugar levels and metabolism.

When boys start producing drastically higher levels of testosterone, they change. They change dramatically. Testosterone affects their brains, not just what they are thinking about but the development of the brain and neuropathways, their genitals change, their muscles change and of course their behavior changes as their internal biochemical mechanics shift into a new gear. Their biology is changing the way they see the world and their place in it. They develop a drive that affects their personality and decision making and their high level of testosterone can make them feel immortal. Testosterone dampens their perception of pain and as well as their emotional sensitivity making men feel powerful and at times invincible. Ask any older man and he will say he wishes he were 25 again. For many men it is a time of feeling a strong vitality and drive that makes life exciting and fun.

When we understand what testosterone does to the body and psyche, we can see how a decline in testosterone can be quite dramatic for the man experiencing it. Instead of feeling invincible and powerful, now he feels more emotionally sensitive which can lead to new feelings of anxiety or depression. His ability to build muscle and feel strength in the body lessens and his sex drive is also affected. The way in which a man interacts with the world changes. He may feel a great loss as these changes occur. Men become aware of the aging process and their own mortality. As their drive declines, they often worry about what life will bring and whether life will have the passions it once had. They also wonder if they will be able to continue to meet the challenges that life will bring. It is quite an intense shift that occurs with declining testosterone.

Testosterone is not just about sex, but sex is a big deal. For many men especially those with higher testosterone levels, the sexual drive and the fulfillment of that drive are critical experiences in their lives. Culturally and physiologically men are tuned to connecting intimately through the physical act of sex. They tend to connect first through physical contact and then open the doors to the heart and emotions. When a man's libido or sexual function declines, he may be at a loss as to how to connect with his partner. When he cannot engage in sex or cannot rely upon his body to perform sexually, he may have lost his tool for connecting. The double whammy of a man not being able to rely upon his body sexually and feeling increased emotional sensitivity from lower testosterone along with his partner's decreased libido, can really do a number on a man's confidence and self-esteem. It is often a big shift for men to find new ways to engage intimately as they go through andropause.

Andropause and menopause give us the opportunity to upgrade our relationships and bring them to the next stage in our lives. No longer is the marriage and partnership primarily focused on creating and maintaining family where each partner's needs are often superseded by the children's and family's needs. Now we can turn to one another as individuals to enjoy each other anew and step through the gateway to the development of a closer and more intimate relationship. It takes courage and willingness to explore new ways of connecting and communicating. In this process our lower level of hormones help us to make this transition. Instead of relying on the strong physical drive of libido, we now call upon our hearts and minds to take the jump into connection and emotional intimacy.

Feeling Good through the Hormonal Change

Now that you have a greater perspective on what is happening within your body and mind as you move through this rite of passage, you can develop daily practices to feel good again! We will discuss practices and health habits as well as supplements and hormones to bring the body back into a high state of health and wellness. Your health needs are changing and what you do on a daily basis can have a great impact either positively or negatively on how you feel. It takes more time and effort to care for the body as we get older but the body also becomes much more efficient so putting good practices in play has dramatic and lasting benefits. Caring for the body pays off!

The more attention you put into engaging in whole body health practices, the less you will need supplements, medicines, or hormones. I have outlined health practices first – practices you can do as part of your daily life to feel good and bring your body to a higher state of health. These practices form the foundation for lifelong wellness. We will tackle the topics of weight gain, food and nutritional needs, movement and exercise – your foundational health practices – and then get into nutritional supplements, herbal medicine, and bioidentical hormone therapy for hormone balance and maintenance.

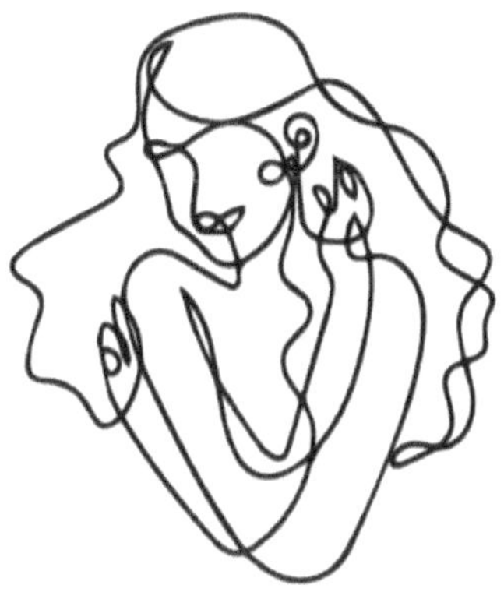

Weight ~ Embracing Your Body

Weight is an uncomfortable topic. As girls most of us experienced many messages about what it meant to be an attractive woman and how our weight played into that equation. From our peers we heard about diets and schemes on losing weight quickly and compared ourselves with the lean figures of models and social media posts, often shunning images of larger women. Parents and coaches also contributed to the formation of our ideal body image which culturally has leaned toward slim bodies and less curves. Throughout their lives, most women do not feel truly at home and comfortable within their bodies. Instead their body receives constant criticism and even hatred for not being perfect. The discomfort and negative judgment so many women have for their bodies only gets compounded during perimenopause.

Weight gain and changes in body shape are laments voiced by many women during perimenopause and into menopause. As a woman's progesterone production decreases, her estrogen becomes dominant causing both weight gain and difficulty losing weight. When her estrogen finally falls, the fat storage she previously carried in her hips and thighs migrates to her waistline, belly, and torso. So even if a woman can maintain her normal weight during perimenopause, her shape will change and not in a way she wants!

Shifting hormones slow her metabolism and often bring it to a screeching halt again contributing to weight gain. It now takes more time, effort, and changes to both eating plans and exercise routines to shed excess pounds. This becomes the perfect storm for many women. On top of being sleep deprived, more emotional, and having hot flashes, she becomes saddled with unwanted weight gain or more fat around her waistline all contributing to her sense of frustration and futility. But there are ways to return to normal weight and feel good in the body again; it just takes dedication, change, and stamina.

It is a worthwhile investment to find our way back to our ideal weight. Not only does it make us feel good about our bodies and ourselves, but it also delivers significant health benefits. Excess fat in our bodies operates as a storage facility for estrogen, hormone disruptor chemicals, and fat-soluble toxins. Shedding excess fat will help maintain better estrogen/progesterone balance and decrease the cancer and disease risks associated with estrogen dominance. Decreasing our fat stores also lowers our chemical load again decreasing chronic disease and cancer risk. The difficult work of weight loss and maintenance truly pays off when we consider long term health.

The billion-dollar diet industry knows we will pay anything for the magic pill to find and maintain our ideal weight. But most women know through experience there is no magic pill or special diet to guarantee weight loss and maintenance for life. It takes consistency, attention, and intention to both the foods we eat and drink and our physical movement to reach our body goals. Getting the endocrine system back on track is often the missing link when a woman cannot maintain her weight with her regular exercise routine and good diet. In fact, no amount of exercise and good eating can help a woman lose weight when her thyroid or sex hormones are significantly out of balance. We have to address the whole picture to reach our weight goals.

On the other side of the equation is low body weight. Women can restrict their eating and consume too few calories or insufficient beneficial fats and nutrients to keep their body weight low. This will also negatively impact a woman's hormone balance. Insufficient body fat will interfere with adequate hormone production and even adding hormones into the treatment plan will be unsuccessful if a woman maintains a body weight that is too low for her frame. She will also be saddled with an increased risk for joint issues and low bone density if her body weight remains too low. For women who had low or normal body weight when they started perimenopause, gaining a small amount of weight during perimenopause and into menopause can be beneficial.

Practice 6 – Making Friends with Your Body

There is no better time to change your relationship with weight than right now. The moment to stop suffering has come. Let's explore some of the juice behind weight issues so we may move forward into a healthier and more loving relationship with our bodies.

How do you feel about your body? Would you say you are friends with your body, foes, or neutral?

In an ideal situation, how would you like to feel about your body? Can you imagine feeling love towards your body? Can you imagine feeling comfortable with your body and not judging it? Take this moment to close your eyes, sit quietly and feel what it would feel like to be friends with your body. Stay with it for a few minutes, really feel throughout your whole body and into your heart what it would feel like to be best friends with your body.

A big part of having a happy relationship with your body is being able to imagine it. We must imagine it before we can live it. We are often caught up in an incessant rant about all the things we hate about our bodies. How can we see anything else when our judgments fill our minds 24/7? We cannot. We need to create space to connect with and begin a friendship with our bodies so our bodies can love us back.

Each day set aside a few minutes – upon waking in the morning and before going to bed each night and visualize what it feels like to live in your ideal body. Make your expectations realistic – if you are 5'2", you are not going to grow to 5'8" but you could feel longer and leaner and thus feel taller. If you are 175 pounds and want to come down to 145 pounds, you will be more successful if you first imagine yourself at 160 pounds then as you near that goal, start to imagine yourself at 150 and then with time 145. Give your body time to adjust. If you want to be able to move your body without pain, first imagine the pain lessened then move to feeling only stiffness. Then as you progress, imagine moving smoothly and freely with happiness and comfort. Start with goals that are a positive step from where you are but not such a big leap that you get frustrated by not meeting that goal quickly. The body will take a little time to adjust and being friends with the body means giving it the time and resources to be successful not to sabotage it.

In your quiet time imagine what this new body feels like. What does it look like? How does it move? If negative thoughts come up during this exercise, let them float away. Let any negative feelings, thoughts, or images fade away during your visualization time. This is precious reprogramming time where you get to connect with what you want. Value it and care for it gently. This is part of creating the next iteration of you.

You can take this exercise a step further by creating a vision board for your new body. Collect images of new clothes you may wear, new hairstyles or makeup you may try, new activities you may engage in as you shift your body into this new place. Let yourself get excited about it. You can even start some of these changes now – get that haircut, try on that new style even before your body gets to your goal. You are investing in yourself and you deserve it!

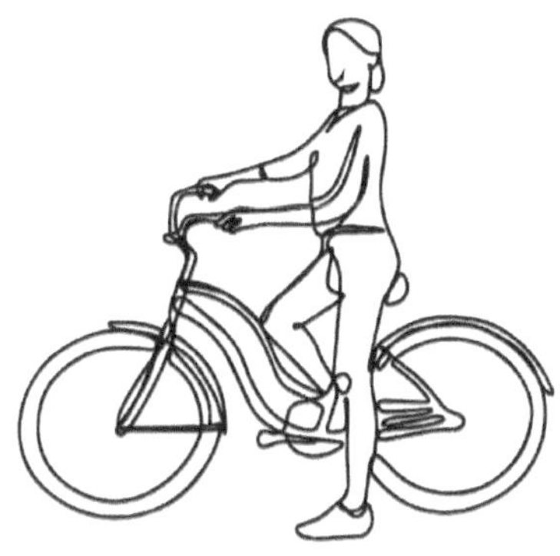

Movement and Exercise

What is the single best activity we can do to feel better during perimenopause? Movement. Exercise gives us energy, helps us manage stress, makes us sleep better, helps the brain function better, manages our weight which makes us feel good and balances our hormones which makes us feel even better. That being said, being underweight and over exercising will make you feel worse and will throw your hormones out of balance even more. Regular exercise supports good health better than almost anything else. We are made to move. No matter how life and technology change, our bodies were still made to be active. There is nothing that will make up for a lack of movement. It is essential just like food and sleep. Find something you like to do or someone you like to do it with and get out and do it!

How to be Successful with Exercise

If you have not developed a regular exercise or movement routine by the time you start perimenopause, there is no time to lose! At this point in life you can have a significant positive impact on your health by making movement a part of your life. Women often say they will exercise more when they retire or when the kids are gone, but if you do not start moving now, it will be harder to move then. This is also the time in your life when exercise will have its greatest impact on your long term health. You can increase heart health and increase bone density in profound ways at this point. In later years it will be more important to maintain heart and brain health and bone density. But the effort you put in now actually changes your risks factors and builds a greater foundation for health. You will need this solid foundation of heart and brain health and strong bones to draw from in the years to come. This is the time of life to deposit into your body's health savings account. Just like the money you put into a retirement account, what you invest now pays off later.

Make It a Routine

Like anything else that is important, you have to make it a priority. The more you move, the more you will be able to move. The less you move, the more pain you will have and more muscle, joint, and bone issues you will have which will end up restricting your movement. The old saying "move or lose it", is relevant here. Develop an exercise routine that becomes a regular part of your life. Your routine can consist of a variety of movement outlets; it does not need to be one sport or an athletic event that you are training for. It does need to consist of activities that are realistic for you or that you can envision yourself doing. Do not sabotage yourself by having goals that would require your super human effort if exercise is already a challenge for you. Choose activities that you are familiar with or curious about. Let yourself consider what may not be comfortable now but with time and practice you may really enjoy. Stretching yourself is good but taking a leap that is more intimidating than inspiring may prevent you from meeting your goals and further undermine your confidence in your body. If there is no exercise or movement that you like to do, find someone you like to spend time with who will commit to exercising with you or a pet who needs to get out and walk regularly. Find a class or center that offers activities that you have been curious about and sign up! Paying money can be a good incentive, you may go to class if you do not want to waste the money you have invested.

Reward Yourself

For those of you who have never been successful with an exercise routine, develop a reward system for yourself. Create a system for yourself where you reward yourself for meeting your exercise goal each time. For daily or weekly activities, make it a small reward or give yourself 'points' each time you complete your exercise and then use those points toward a larger reward. Find rewards other than food! If food is your reward, you will find yourself not meeting your weight goals and feeling sabotaged all over again. Rewards can range from activities like taking a bath with special bath salts, watching a show you like but do not usually have time for, taking time to enjoy music you love without doing anything else, saving up for clothing or make up that you have your eyes on, collecting images of places you would like to visit and making a small contribution to your travel fund each time you exercise. When you reward yourself for creating a new health habit you get two-fold benefit – loving your healthier body and investing in your heart's desires! The joy and satisfaction that come from investing in yourself continue to build. As you get used to feeling good in your body, you want to keep it going. It feels wonderful to have energy, to be able to move freely, and feel good in your skin. You will want to keep up your new exercise habits just to keep feeling this way. When you fall off your routine and the old aches and pains and lethargy find their way back into your body, you know you can turn it around. You have before! Each time you get back into the routine of caring for yourself, you will want to keep it going because it feels so good! Vitality becomes its own reward.

Changing Up Your Routine

Women who have exercised regularly for years before perimenopause often find that their old routines no longer work for them. They have more joint achiness or fatigue. Their blood pressure changes, or they feel out of breath more easily. Body pain or muscle spasms keep them from being able to perform their old standby routines. The body is signaling a need for change. Listening to your body signals will allow you to continue to be active without injuring yourself and then needing to take time off to recover. Women who have previously done high intensity cardiovascular exercise may need to dial down the high impact until their hormones are balanced. Perimenopausal sleep problems and frequent hot flashes can deplete a woman requiring her to moderate her exercise if only temporarily. If a woman continues to push herself and ignore her body's signals, she will deplete herself further and worsen her hormone imbalance. Recovery will take longer and all her hard work will end in frustration and fatigue.

Try these exercise hacks if your old workouts are making you feel worse instead of better. Run or cycle at a more moderate intensity or do high intensity bursts for a shorter period of time. Shift from high impact exercises like running and step aerobics to spin classes and moderate impact dance or cardio classes. Run on a track, sand, or dirt instead of pavement or sidewalks. Move into cross training to avoid repetitive stress to one part of the body. Move to more varied routines and listen to your body's response. Instead of pushing with the mind, listen more to the body. When it gives you feedback that an exercise is painful during or after the workout, change it up. Lower hormone levels can cause problems with bladder leakage and uterine or bladder prolapse during high impact activities. Switching to more moderate or low impact activities with high cardiovascular intensity can keep the endorphins up without stressing the bladder and uterus.

Over time the body becomes more efficient and will eventually burn less calories doing the same workout. To increase your metabolism, you must change up your routine. Try interval training - bursts of higher intensity or faster cardio movements intermixed with slower movements. The change itself from slow to fast movements requires the body to burn more fuel and gets excess fat stores burning. You may need to increase your workout times or vary your workouts between short strength building sessions and longer cardiovascular sessions. Incorporate more hills or stairs into your walks; do shorter workouts more frequently; try dividing your longer workout into two shorter sessions on the same day. Balance your ashtanga yoga routine with hatha routines and yin yoga. Variety and change will be the winning combinations at this juncture to keep fat stores down in the normal range.

This is the time to build bone. You need to be holding the body weight during exercise to stimulate the bones to build and maintain their strength. If you swim or bike, take a few days each week to walk or do weight training exercises. Balance out weight bearing with your non weight bearing activities. If you have smaller bones or are lighter weight, add a backpack or weights during your walks or hikes. Increasing the amount of weight your body is carrying will increase your bone strength and promote stronger bones long term.

The shifting needs of your body now include more attention to joint health. The effects of gravity and the physical work of our lives start to show up in knee pain, hip pain, sciatic pain, back pain, plantar fasciitis and frozen shoulders. We are tempted to move less when our body hurts, but the body may be signaling us to move differently. We often need to focus more on strengthening and stretching the body at this point instead of pushing for cardiovascular effort. Our core muscles need constant strengthening to support both the muscles and the bones in our backs. Knee and hip pain often reflect problems with dysfunctional movement. Our alignment is off, and we are stressing some muscles too much and others not enough resulting in joint pain from misalignment. Have your posture and movement assessed by a knowledgeable physical therapist, chiropractor, or sports trainer. Correcting body positioning now can save you years of pain. Chronic inflammation that shows up in plantar fasciitis and frozen shoulders can alert us to systemic issues with inflammation. It is time to look at the body as a whole and see what is contributing to this inflammation as well as developing health routines that clear inflammation and promote a greater range of movement.

Working with the body to help it feel good again and increase its ease of movement is a great investment in your future health and happiness. When you take the time to care for your body, you are committing to your wellness and making the statement that you are worth care and attention. You are telling yourself you deserve your own love and care. You have given it to others for so much of your life – now it is your time!

Practice 7 – Making Exercise Work for You

When a woman loves her body, she wants to move it. It feels good to move and feel at home in the body. But when a woman is saddled with extra weight that she feels ashamed of or a body she hates, movement does not feel good. If a woman has had injuries or is limited in her mobility, it may also be difficult to move the way she desires. We want to find ways to move the body that support agility, strength, balance and lifelong health.

If exercise has been difficult for you in the past, now is the perfect time to let it go and move on. Today we can focus on our path to success and every little step that moves us closer. We are going to formulate a movement program that is personalized for you and contains the components needed for long term success. An exercise program is another investment in yourself and your happiness.

Here are a list of activities to get you thinking about all types of movement that you can include in your personalized program. What interests you? What have you always wanted to try? What would you secretly love to be able to do? Once you have determined a few activities that call to you, we will create a weekly routine that fits into your life and can be easily maintained.

Walk	Bike
Hike	Swim
Water aerobics	Surfing
Golf	Badminton
Racquetball	Pickle ball
Tennis	Stationary bike
Elliptical machine	Skating
Ice skating	Skiing
Snow shoeing	Weightlifting
Rubber band workout	Pilates
Yoga	Karate
Tai Chi	Aikido
Dancing	Gardening
Housecleaning	Washing the car
Walk or bike when running errands	
Mowing the lawn	Kayaking
Row machine	Boxing
Roller derby	Hockey
Basketball	Running

I. What 3 physical activities do you enjoy or could see yourself doing:

1.
2.
3.

II. Go through your weekly calendar or schedule. Find 4 time slots where you could fit in movement. If you are not exercising currently, this can be 20 minutes to start with. If you have been exercising, make it 30-45-minute time slot.

1.
2.
3.
4.

An exercise schedule can look like this:
For women who are just getting started:
Option A
Monday – walk or stationary bike at lunch or after work (20-30 minutes)
Tuesday – stretch at home after work (20 minutes)
Thursday – gym or walk before work or at lunch (20- 30minutes)
Saturday – take the dog for a longer walk (30 minutes)

Option B
Tuesday and Thursday – walk after work (20-30 minutes)
Wednesday and Saturday– Pilates class (DVD or download from youtube) (20-30 minutes)

Option C
Saturday and Sunday – walk in community pool or water aerobics class (30 minutes
Tuesday and Thursday – ride stationary bike at home or at your local YMCA (20-30 minutes)

For women who want to kick it up a notch:
Option A
Monday, Wednesday – gym workout, cardiovascular (30-45 minutes)
Tuesday, Thursday – strength workout (20 -30 minutes)
Saturday – stretch, walk, or yard work

Option B
Tuesday and Thursday – swim in pool (30 minutes+)
Wednesday – stretch (20-30 minutes)
Saturday and Sunday – hike, take a long walk, play pickle ball (45-60+ minutes)

Option C
Monday and Wednesday – yoga DVD at home (30-40 minutes)
Tuesday and Thursday – elliptical or treadmill (30 minutes)
Saturday – walk with a friend (45+ minutes)

For women who are serious about weight loss:
Option A
Monday and Wednesday – cardiovascular (kick boxing, step aerobics, Zumba, spin class) (45-60 minutes)
Tuesday and Thursday – combo weights and stretching (30-45 minutes)
Saturday – hike, bike, long walk, water activity (45+ minutes)

Option B
Monday and Wednesday – more moderate cardio (dance, treadmill, elliptical) (50-60 minutes)
Thursday – yoga, Pilates (50-60 minutes)
Saturday – bike (45 minutes+)
Sunday – weights, Pilates (30 minutes)

III. Create a colorful calendar or find an app for your phone where you can schedule in movement times, set your alarm, or have notifications sent to remind you.

Put your exercise clothes in the car before you go to work. Carry walking shoes with you or leave them at the office for walks during your lunch or breaks. Exercise on your way to work by riding your bike, walking to the bus, or walking to your carpool pick up point. Turn in your high heels for shoes that could be used for walking during the day. Change up your wardrobe a few days a week to allow for lunchtime walks or walking to meetings instead of driving.

IV. Motivation Hacks

Somedays it is difficult to exercise – you feel tired, you are super busy, you have a headache or you could think of five other things you would prefer doing. Just remember this is your life. Invest in yourself. Sitting down and watching TV or reaching for that glass of wine will not make you feel better tomorrow. You will be disappointed in yourself for letting yourself down. You have a plan to feel better – stick with it! You will see that following your routine will make you feel better. The energy will come. Happiness will again flow through your body. Keep your goal in mind and commit! You deserve it!

Here are some motivation hacks to keep you moving forward even when it feels like you are slipping backward. Putting these strategies into your exercise plan will make it easier and often more fun as you reach your goal.

Find a reliable exercise buddy – neighbor, friend, co-worker

Hire an exercise coach

Join an exercise group – boot camp, weight loss training class, fundraising organizations that do walks, 5K's, bike rides

Walk your dog or borrow a friend's or neighbor's dog that needs some extra walking

Reward yourself for meeting your goals especially at the beginning of your routine before you start to see your body changing (have the reward be something other than food)

Therapy can help. When your plans keep falling through or you see that you are sabotaging yourself, seek out a helping hand. Body image issues and having difficulty sticking with a self-care plan can be related to emotional or psychological blocks. We all have blocks somewhere in our lives. If you see a pattern where you keep sabotaging yourself or cannot follow through on a program that you know would help, hire an expert to assist you in discovering and clearing away roadblocks to your success. Then you will be free to go back to the drawing board and try again, this time successfully!

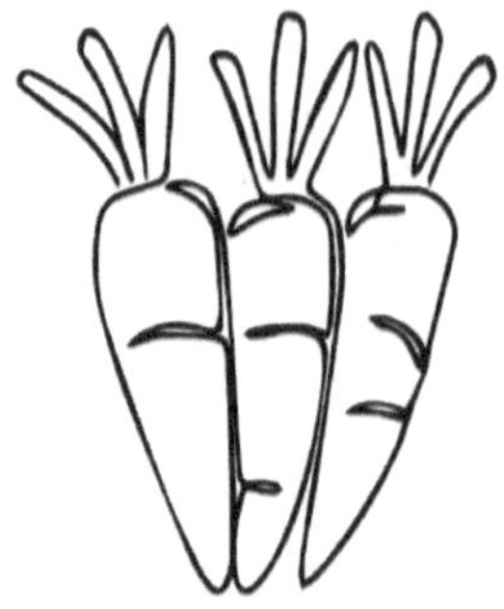

Food ~ Love, Nourishment, and Nutrition

Food is an integral part of our daily lives serving as both physical sustenance and pleasure. Is it any wonder that food is such a rich topic throughout our lives? Food is our body's fuel and has a huge impact on our health. It can help us by increasing energy, supporting a positive, uplifted mood, balancing blood sugar and stimulating mental activity; or it can harm us by interfering with sleep, increasing mood swings, draining our energy and making our joints achy. It is our choice how we use food and if we want to make it work for us rather than against us. We have access to any food we want all year round. Gone are the days of seasonal foods and seasonal changes to our diet. And though it is wonderful to have such constant access to wonderful food, it is also a challenge to moderate it. We can eat what we want when we want it, and we do not always make the connection between what we are putting in our mouths and how we will feel later. Our relationship with food is a complex one and if we honor that complexity, we can make the adjustments we need to feel better as we move through perimenopause.

During her fertile years, a woman needs higher levels of nutrients, fats, and carbohydrates to maintain her monthly menstrual cycle and replenish her ability to conceive. Supporting a woman's menstrual cycle is an energy intensive process requiring additional calories and specific nutrients to keep the system operating strongly. As a woman transitions into menopause, she will find she often has less tolerance for her previous diet. The same foods that nurtured her before now start to cause digestive upset, weight gain, or blood sugar imbalances. Her appetite will often decrease even if she continues the same amount of exercise. The body is giving her the message that it is changing and has new needs. It is time for a diet overhaul.

Adjusting our diets to include a greater variety and higher percentage of vegetables, a smaller amount of lean animal proteins and more plant based proteins and a smaller portion of grains will help us move into the menopausal years feeling good in our bodies without the excess weight we dread. In my practice I see many women naturally gravitating toward new diets as they go through menopause. When their children grow up and leave home, moms find it to be a good time to try new eating plans. Many couples find they do not need as much protein or grains to feel satisfied, and they feel more energetic without them. They find they sleep better and have less digestive upset with including more vegetables and eating smaller portions overall.

Both our immune system and digestive system change in perimenopause. We see more gas, bloating, and constipation when eating grains or larger portions of meat and an increase in food allergy or sensitivity reactions. The body is signaling us to change our routine. It is time to upgrade our eating habits to support this new body that is being created. Experimenting with new food plans can give us the feedback we need to see what our bodies like and which fuels support them best.

Changing Nutrient Needs

In this section we will go through what our bodies need in perimenopause and beyond. I have broken each major nutrient into sections and then will examine specific food plans.

Grains and Carb's

Carbohydrates are one the main fuels we get from food. They are found in sugars, starches, and fibers from fruits, grains, vegetables and milk products. Carbohydrates play an important role in the proper functioning of our bodies, but we tend to overconsume them because they are satisfying and taste good. Though carbohydrates come from whole foods naturally, overconsumption is more of a problem when we eat more processed than whole foods. When we get most of our carbohydrates from vegetables and beans, we naturally limit the amount we eat because their high fiber content makes them filling and slow to digest.

When we are feeding a baby during pregnancy or supporting a monthly reproductive cycle, we need carbohydrates and grains. The nutrients from whole grains and carbohydrates help us produce sufficient hormones and keep us cycling regularly. But when reproduction winds down and our body needs change, we no longer digest carbohydrates well. At this point excess carbohydrates turn to fat in our bodies and increase triglyceride and cholesterol levels. Our hormonal changes make us less tolerant of grains and starches.

This is a great time to experiment with carbohydrates. Grains and starches are satisfying and comforting so including a small amount of them in the diet or finding alternatives to them are important. Cauliflower rice instead of white rice, zucchini noodles instead of wheat noodles and lettuce wraps instead of bread or tortillas are all examples of how we can switch from grains to vegetables and still enjoy our favorite meals without a big carb load. Instead of sandwiches try colorful salads with candied winter squash for a carb satisfier. Try veggie chips instead of tortilla chips with salsa or hummus. Include carrot, squash, or quinoa noodles with a spinach pesto sauce instead of wheat pasta. Finding ways to decrease the amount of carbohydrates in your favorite meals will make them more satisfying in the end because you will still get the flavor you are looking for without the bloating and gas that weigh you down. Eating without grains has never been easier. Many parents find that as their children grow up and leave home, they naturally shift meals to incorporating more vegetables and less heavy grains. Their growing teenagers are not there anymore with their high needs for carbohydrates and proteins. Now parents can shift toward a diet that will support their health and wellbeing for years to come.

Fat Equals Flavor

Fats from plant sources become our faithful friends in menopause. Just as our needs for and tolerance of carbohydrates shift in perimenopause so do our needs for fat. At this time of life plant sources of fat support and nourish the body more than the fats from meat and cow milk products. Avocados, olives, flax and chia seeds are all examples of plant-based fats that nourish our skin, eyes, digestive and vaginal tracts. Nuts and seeds such as sesame seeds, almonds, walnuts and hazelnuts contribute as well. We want to shift away from animal fats that can increase cholesterol levels while maintaining heart, brain, and joint function with fish and plant-based fats.

When we feel extra pounds building up, we tend to shy away from fat. Fat has more calories per gram than carbohydrates and proteins so it makes logical sense that we could decrease this macronutrient when trying to lose weight. But we need to be more discriminating when it comes to cutting back on fats. Fat itself is necessary for our health but its benefits vary depending on what type it is and where it comes from. Beneficial fats are needed to make hormones so including good fats in our diets supports a balanced and full functioning endocrine system. Plus, fats make food taste good!

Fish and plant-based fats are needed for maintaining brain function in babies as well as in adults. They are also needed for joint health, keeping them flexible and lubricated and keeping arthritis in check. Good fats are found in avocados, fatty fish like salmon, tuna, sardines and anchovies. Olives and olive oil provide nourishment to our tissues along with sesame seeds, almonds, walnuts, pecans, macadamia nuts and sunflower seeds. Plant based oils like evening primrose oil, borage oil, and black currant oil support normal hormone production from the fertile years to menopause. The fats we want to minimize are those from animal sources, fried foods, fat for cow milk products and the oils from corn, soy, and cottonseed. Reach for salad dressings with olive oil or tahini instead of ranch, thousand island or milk based creamy dressings. Instead of cheese as a condiment reach for avocados or olives. Put a nut butter based sauce over vegetables instead of butter. It is easy to find fun, delicious recipes online to discover new food loves.

Plant vs. Animal Protein

Our need for protein significantly changes over our lifetimes. During childhood and adolescence, we need significant amounts of protein to build bones, muscles, and develop our immune system. During pregnancy and lactation, we also have high protein needs to meet the demands of our growing baby. But when our fertility decreases, and we no longer have regular periods our protein needs lessen. We still need protein but in much smaller quantities than in earlier years. New diet trends run the gamut from solely plant-based diets on one side and to high animal-based protein diets on the other. Some people will thrive on a hundred percent plant-based diet naturally lower in protein while others will feel their best on a higher animal protein diet. It is important to learn which proteins you digest better and which support your energy and vitality. For some people smaller amounts of animal proteins will support long term muscle, bone, and heart health while others will thrive on purely plant based proteins such as beans, sprouted grains, quinoa, nuts and seeds, tofu and green pea protein. Protein helps us balance blood sugar levels so knowing how plant and animal proteins affect your blood sugar balance and energy are important in determining your specific optimal diet.

Experimenting with New Eating Plans

Food plans and diets go through trends just like the fashion industry. Every five to seven years a new diet appears promising to be the diet to end all diets, the magic ticket to make all of our body image dreams come true. Do you remember the old grapefruit for breakfast Stewardess Diet of the 1970's or the hugely popular Atkins and Palm Beach Diet of the 1980's and 90's? The hippy movement turned to vegetarianism, whole grains, and soy protein during the 1970's and 80's. The new millennia witnessed the rise of the Paleo Diet, Mediterranean Diet and Blood Type Diet. Currently in vogue are Intermittent Fasting, the Whole 30, DASH and the resurrection of the Keto Diet. Nutrition education is also continuously changing as evidenced by the old food industry designed 4 Food Groups taught in public schools in the 1970's and 80's to the redesigned Food Pyramid of the 1990's and now the current My Plate model. We cannot agree on what makes a healthy diet even with an immense amount of data around nutrition, disease development and progression. How do you sort through all the conflicting information on food and find what is right for you?

Over my 30 years of studying nutrition and diets I have discovered that there is no single perfect diet for everyone, and there is no one truth about nutrition. There are, however, reemerging themes and data that elucidate what keeps most people healthy over their lifetimes. We know that too many carbohydrates are not beneficial after menopause, and we do not want to replace protein with more carbohydrates. We know that some protein is important as we age but it may be individual variation that determines whether that be entirely plant-based protein or a combination of animal and plant-based protein. Vegetables never get bad press in health research, but for some with digestive issues, cooking vegetables may be more beneficial than a purely raw vegetable diet or a large percentage of juiced vegetables. For others with compromised absorption, juicing and raw vegetables can provide wonderful nourishment.

How do you determine which diet is best for you? Experiment! With the wealth of resources, we have these days from books, food blogs, cookbooks and internet recipes from all over the world, we can easily experiment with different food plans and evaluate what makes us feel the best. Choose a food plan that interests you then follow it for at least 30 days. If you are feeling good on that plan, give it a three-month trial run. The body will continue to change and adapt to the new diet over those three months and will give you plenty of feedback about how that plan affects your energy, digestion, and whole body health. When you find a plan that makes you feel good, you will want to stay with it. Even when you fall off your plan, you will want to return to it when you are ready. Many of my patients follow the Whole30 Plan every January as a reset, a way to get back on track with their eating and get off the sugar and food binge of holiday time.

The Super Nutrients: Minerals and Antioxidants

In perimenopause and beyond our needs increase for specific nutrients especially for minerals and antioxidants. Antioxidants protect us from environmental factors that accelerate the aging process and increase the risk for cancer. Minerals are crucial for tissue and bone repair and are needed in greater amounts when our production of bone and tissues slow in menopause. Minerals also support heart rhythm function, nerve conduction, and glandular functioning. We have come to a place in life where we need fewer total calories each day but more specific nutrients so nutrient rich foods become the key to a lifelong health.

Antioxidants

You have probably heard about antioxidants, but you may not know what they do in the body and why they are so important for slowing the aging process and maintaining long term health. Antioxidants are naturally occurring biochemicals found in foods that can protect cells from damage. When cells are protected from early oxidation or too much oxidation, the aging process is slowed. Cells are healthier for longer and can continue to do their work of supporting the body. The reverse of this, too much oxidation, promotes inflammation in the body through cellular breakdown. Keeping oxidation low by including antioxidant foods is another significant factor in keeping inflammation in check.

Antioxidants support heart vessel, eye, and skin health. We are constantly exposed to factors in our environment that cause oxidation such as sun exposure, smoking, and environmental toxins. Eating foods that are fried, smoked, or grilled also increase our oxidative load just as infections and psychological stress do.

The older we get the more we need the antioxidants from fruit and vegetables to support us. In nature most of our antioxidants come from fruit. Nature gives us a visual clue about antioxidant rich fruits through their color. The orange of mangos, apricots, and cantaloupe give us a clue of their carotenoid content. The red of tomatoes and red bell peppers show off their lycopene content. The blues and purples in blue berries, raspberries, and black berries give away their proanthocyanadin content. Nature speaks to us through color and presents us a pleasing visual spectrum of what foods to include in our diets for optimum health. Eating a variety of fruits and vegetables from different spectrums of the rainbow gives us a comprehensive mix of antioxidants and nutrients.

Research on antioxidants has been robust over the last twenty years giving rise to increased knowledge and availability of super foods. These super foods are nutrient dense and full of antioxidants giving us an opportunity to receive a wide variety of health benefits from specific foods. Super foods include all the dark-skinned berries – raspberries, blackberries, blueberries - dark skinned grapes, kale, Brussel sprouts and other cruciferous vegetables, tomatoes, acai, maca and more! From smoothies and revamped restaurant menus to nutritional supplements, these foods are finding their way into our lives greatly enhancing our cell regeneration and decreasing our risk for disease.

Appendix A in the back of the book provides a thorough list of antioxidants from the carotenoids (including lutein, lycopene and zeaxanthin) to the flavonoids (quercetin, catechins, and isoflavones) and their specific health benefits.

Minerals

Minerals are also needed in greater amounts in menopause. Our bones, teeth, skin, hair and thyroid all need significant amounts of minerals to stay strong and regenerate. Bone loss occurs more rapidly after menopause due to the lower amounts of sex hormones so mineral needs increase. Exercise stimulates the body to deposit these minerals into the bones, creating stronger, denser bones. But without the stimulus of exercise or weight bearing activities, the body will not deposit the minerals into the bones. Every cell in our body uses minerals for its daily functions so we need to provide minerals regularly either through our diets or nutritional supplements. We once received minerals in our water, but modern filtration practices pull the minerals out of our water. Vegetables, whole grains, and fruit also had higher mineral content historically, but erosion and farming practices have depleted minerals from the soil and thus from our foods. The oceans now have a higher mineral content, and we can use this to our advantage by including sea vegetables into our diets. Adding dried seaweed to anything we cook in water, remineralizes our food and gives it a mild salty flavor. You can add seaweed when making soups, beans, stews, rice or other grains. Sea salt, dulse, and other seaweeds can also be sprinkled onto food at mealtime adding a rich flavor while also providing key minerals.

Vegetables continue to be our greatest food source of minerals. Green leafy vegetables provide the minerals calcium and iron while root vegetables provide potassium and phosphorus. Cruciferous vegetables such as broccoli, kale, and Brussel sprouts provide many cancer fighting nutrients as well as calcium, magnesium, and selenium. Vegetables also provide our best sources of vitamins and fiber. Eating vegetables with their natural fibers instead of drinking their juice keeps our digestive tract moving along. A plant-based diet can meet the majority of our mineral and vitamin needs without having to rely upon supplements.

The most important minerals are included here with the minor players included in Appendix B in the back of the book.

We have all heard about **calcium**, the most abundant of the minerals and its key role in bone, teeth, and nail formation. Calcium is less well known for its importance in buffering the blood stream for normal cell function; clotting the blood after a bleeding injury; and maintaining normal heart action and muscle contraction.

Calcium is found in a great variety of foods including green leafy vegetables such as spinach, kale, broccoli and cabbage as well as sesame and chia seeds, almonds, canned sardines and salmon, and some beans including soybeans. Though cow milk products are high in calcium they do not end up depositing much calcium into the bones. Milk products are acid forming which requires pulling calcium out of the bones and into the blood stream to buffer the acidity. At the end of the equation, cow milk products do not end up helping our bone density as much as we once thought.

Magnesium is a crucial mineral that is often deficient in our diets. Magnesium is a powerhouse of a mineral and one of my personal favorites. It is needed in more than 300 biochemical reactions in the body including the initiation and regulation of nerve conduction, releasing muscle contractions, producing thyroid hormones, maintaining bone density and supporting both electrical and mechanical heart function.

Magnesium is found in nuts and seeds (especially walnut and almonds), legumes, whole grains, dark leafy greens including spinach, bananas, fish, dark chocolate and avocadoes.

Zinc is another major player in maintaining the health and normal functioning of the body. It is a major component of the immune system and thyroid hormones. It is needed for the formation of bones, teeth and hair. It regulates blood sugar and supports wound healing. **Good sources of zinc** are nuts and seeds especially pepita pumpkin seeds; shellfish, whole grains, meat and eggs.

Selenium's role in health has come to light much more in the last twenty years. It is needed for normal function of the immune system especially in preventing cancer; it is an integral part of thyroid hormone production and important in maintaining prostate health. Food sources of selenium include Brazil nuts, seeds, fish and green vegetables.

Practice 8 – Nourishment

Let's approach finding a new eating plan or making changes to your current diet with an attitude of curiosity instead of one of deprivation. Our goal is to develop a way of eating that supports your energy, tissue repair, health and longevity while also tasting good! Instead of staying with your same old diet, let's make mealtime more creative and introduce foods that provide significant nutrients making you feel better even after mealtime.

What diets have you been curious about?

What diets have you tried before that worked well and made you feel good but you did not stick with long term? What made it difficult to stay with that diet?

What do you eat that you know your body does not like?

Choose a food plan that interests you and looks realistic for you. Try that plan for 30 days. Instead of bemoaning what you cannot eat during that month, get interested in new recipes and keep in tune with how your body is responding. The more committed you are to following your new plan during the month, the easier you will be able to see results. You can decide at the end of the month how that plan worked for you and if you want to continue it. You are in charge. No one else is determining what you can and cannot eat. You are engaging in a deeper relationship with the body. See where it goes.

Journal about what feelings come up for you as you try new foods. Record changes in your symptoms: nasal or sinus congestion, changes in bowel movements, upset stomach, gas, bloating, headaches or mood changes. What symptoms were you having regularly before new the 30-day diet? How are your symptoms changing during the 30 days? When you reintroduce your old foods back into your diet after the 30 days, do some old symptoms return or worsen that had been gone during the month? Avoid focusing on weight during the first 30 days. Your weight will not change much or at all in those first 30 days.

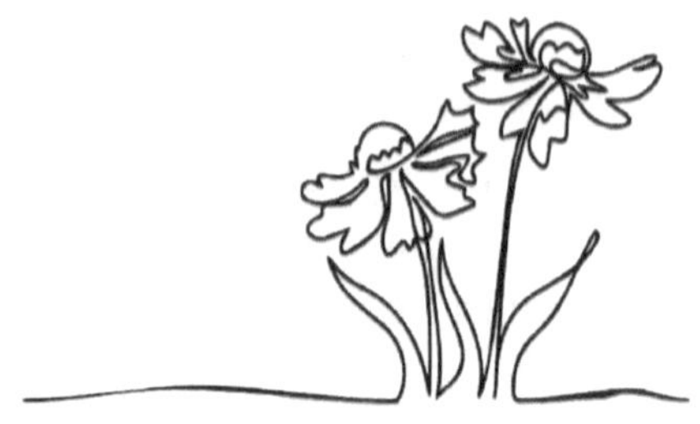

Herbal Medicine ~ The Natural Way to Hormone Balance

Medicine from plants was our first medicine on Earth and even today continues to play a significant role in health and healing. In the context of perimenopausal and menopausal symptoms, herbal medicine can directly assist our bodies in the production of hormones as well as supporting systems in the body that are impacted by hormone imbalance. In early menopause herbal medicine can improve hormone production by decreasing the factors that inhibit hormone production and stimulating glands to increase production. Specific herbs are used to directly target hormone production in the ovaries and adrenal glands during perimenopause. However once a woman reaches menopause, we cannot significantly increase hormone production, but we can support the systems affected by low hormones such as the nervous system, cardiovascular system, and digestive tract. Instead of just managing symptoms with herbal medicine, we focus on improving function of the body systems aiming to prevent recurrence of symptoms in the future. Herbal medicine is a great first line of treatment for hormone imbalance due to its safety and efficacy. It can provide a smoother and more comfortable shift into menopause.

Herbal medicine has been used since the first humans began eating plants in their environment. Historically we would have consumed herbs as part of our diet, gathering fresh herbs for meat and vegetable dishes. Herbs added flavor to foods and helped with food preservation. They were used in both fresh and dried forms and were also consumed as teas. We also indirectly consumed herbs by eating animals that had fed on herbs as they grazed in their natural environment. Even grass-fed cattle today do not have the opportunity to graze on the diversity of herbs that would have been present generations ago. The herbal extracts we use today are more concentrated than what we would have consumed as food generations ago.

My top three favorite herbs for hormone balance are Chaste tree, Maca root, and Black cohosh. Chaste tree and Black cohosh have been used for hundreds of years for hormonal issues while Maca root has been used in South America for millennia. Chaste tree works with the ovaries to enhance progesterone production. Chaste tree can only support the body in making a normal amount of progesterone; it cannot push the body into making excess progesterone, so it has excellent safety. Black cohosh works on the estrogen side of the equation. Often not needed until later in the perimenopausal shift, Black cohosh can help with vaginal dryness, sleep problems, and mild depression associated with low estrogen. It cannot cause the body to make too much estrogen. Maca root has been used for girls, women, and men to address infertility, low libido, low energy, hot flashes and male erectile dysfunction. Maca supports the production of the full line of sex hormones and adrenal hormones. Because Maca can impact the whole range of hormones, it is not appropriate for certain conditions such as androgen dominance or polycystic ovary syndrome.

Herbs such as Lemon balm, Motherwort, Nettles, Milky oats, Skullcap and Linden can be used for perimenopause and menopause related symptoms without affecting hormone levels. Lemon balm and Motherwort are herbs that work with the nervous system and heart to calm heart palpitations and heart rhythm irregularities that are worsened by hormone imbalance. Nettles and Milky oats are nutrient dense herbs supporting mineral needs for hair growth, bone and skin health. Skullcap and Linden can help women sleep better and calm the anxiety they so often feel during perimenopause. I find that using a combination of herbs to directly impact the hormone receptors while also managing the secondary effects of hormone imbalance can be highly effective. Herbal medicine is also remarkably effective in helping younger women return to regular menstrual cycles and decrease PMS symptoms. Herbal medicine, unlike pharmaceuticals, can be tailored to fit an individual's needs. Working with a practitioner well versed in herbal medicine provides women with safe, effective treatments for all phases of hormone change from PMS and irregular cycles to perimenopause and menopause.

Forms of Herbal Medicine

Herbal medicine comes in many forms. The most effective and potent are liquid extracts called tinctures or glycerites. These are extracts from fresh or dried herbs that are preserved with alcohol (tinctures) or glycerin (glycerites). They are potent, cost effective, and easy to use. The downside to tinctures is that they often do not taste good especially the herbs that have the greatest effects on hormone balance. Glycerites taste better due to their sugar content, but not all herbs can be extracted in a glycerin form. Due to the strong taste, some women prefer capsules over liquid tincture or glycerite extracts.

Capsules are wonderful preparations due to their ease of use and lack of negative taste, but they vary greatly in how they are processed and how effective they are. Herbal medicine demands high quality. Particularly when using capsules, I recommend using high quality herbal medicine brands to ensure the formulation will be effective. Herbal teas or infusions can also be used and can be pleasant to include in your daily routine. They tend to be the least potent and most time consuming to prepare, but they are a wonderful way of making your own medicine and healing yourself.

Herbal medicine is also important for its plant-based oils. Flaxseeds, Evening Primrose, Black currant seeds and Borage are four plants whose essential fatty acid constituents are highly beneficial for the endocrine system. These herbs which are often consumed as food work with the endocrine system to enhance hormone production and balance. They can be used as part of the diet by adding them to food or taken as a supplement in capsule or liquid form. These are often the first tools I will use for addressing hormone issues in menstruating, perimenopausal, and post-menopausal women.

Aromatherapy and Essential Oils

The last ten years have seen a dramatic increase in the use of essential oils. These highly potent extracts from plants can be used to assist in many conditions but work very differently from herbs in their whole plant form. Essential oils are highly volatile and are released into the air and dissipate rapidly. Their scent reaches the brain quickly and impacts the limbic system in the forebrain. Though essential oils have some of the same chemical constituents as whole plant extracts, their main effect is on the brain itself. This potent medicine can impact our hormones by stimulating the brain instead of the individual glands themselves. While they can be a great adjunct to therapy, helping with the secondary effects of hormone imbalance such as sleep problems, irritability, fatigue, depression, I do not find that they have a substantial impact for women who are truly low in hormones. They are better used in the early phases of perimenopause instead of later in menopause when hormone levels are low.

Essential oils are best used in modalities that allow them to be smelled to stimulate the limbic portion of the brain. They can be used in diffusers, added to carrier oils for topical use, or mixed with water in spray bottles. Aromatherapy diffusers are containers that have a reservoir to hold a small amount of essential oil. The oils are then either heated by a candle or with an electric or battery powered diffuser, the oil molecules are vibrated to disperse them into the air. Essential oils added to a neutral carrier oil can be massaged into the skin or added to baths. Essential oils can also be mixed with water and used in spray bottles to spray bedding or clothing or as a facial spritzer. Oral ingestion has not proven to be safe and can irritate people with allergies or sensitivities. Because of their potency, essential oils are best used for symptom relief instead of long term daily use.

Practice 9 – Creating Your Own Medicine

Part of empowering yourself through the menopause is creating your own unique wellness plan and making your own medicine to enhance your health and wellbeing now and for years to come. When you put your own energy into your healing, it becomes even more powerful and beneficial. You become your own healer! Herbal medicine is a great tool for creating your own personalized home remedies through using herbs in cooking, teas, and aromatherapy preparations.

Making Your Own Herbal Tea

Herbal teas are both enjoyable to drink as well as beneficial for conditions such as intestinal gas and stomach upset, sleep issues, and anxiety. Try Fennel seed tea with Ginger root or Cardamom seeds for gas or slow digestion. For a calming tea, use Holy Basil leaf (Tulsi), Lemon balm leaf, Milky Oats straw or Lavender flowers. To help with winding down to sleep, a combination of Skullcap flowers, leaves, and stems, Lemonbalm leaf, and Passionflower flowers can be used.

Tea Preparation

When making your own herbal teas, consider which part of the herb or plant you are using. For soft parts such as flowers, leaves, and stems, use 1 Tbsp dried herbs per 1 cup of water. Bring the water to a boil and then take it off the heat. Pour water over herbs in a glass or ceramic container and let steep with a lid on for 15-20 minutes, strain the tea then drink warm or cold. When you are using the hard parts of the plant such as seeds, roots, or bark, use 1 tsp of dried herbs per 1 cup of water. In a glass or ceramic pan, simmer the herbs in the water for 15-20 minutes. Then strain the tea and allow to cool. You can store your tea for a few days in the refrigerator. Limit herbal teas to 3 cups per day.

Herbs in Cooking

Herbs such as Ginger root and Turmeric root can be used in cooking to aid digestion and help calm inflammation. In Ayurvedic medicine Ginger and Turmeric are made into a paste often with coconut oil to retain the medicinal constituents in the herbs. This paste is then used in cooking to impart both flavor and health benefits. Cinnamon can be used for blood sugar control and tastes delicious added to oatmeal, smoothies, and apple dishes. Garlic not only adds its unique flavor to Mediterranean dishes, but it is also one of the best anti-viral agents of all time. Flaxseeds used in smoothies, added to yogurt or cereal, or mixed into salad dressings help with regular bowel movements as well as providing moisture to skin and eyes.

What herbs can you add to your diet to enhance your health? Consider experimenting with Ayurvedic dishes, Mediterranean herbs and spices, or making health booster smoothies to enrich your diet and support wellness.

Aromatherapy

Our sense of smell had a direct pathway to the brain, and this is where aromatherapy has its impact. Scents can bring us deep sensual pleasure making experimentation with essential oils so much fun!

When creating your own aromatherapy blend make sure you are working with high quality essential oils to avoid the harsh chemicals used to extract essential oils in low quality brands. High quality essential oils and carrier oils will yield a formula that both smells good and bestows health benefits.

What type of formula would you like to create – an oil for the bath, a blend to use topically on the skin, a mix to use in a diffuser or a spray for yourself or your room? What symptom do you most want to treat – sleep issues, low energy and mood, stress and anxiety? Try one of these blends below or make a trip to your local health food store and sample the essential oils there; then create your own blend!

Essential oils for energy and mood support: Neroli, Grapefruit, Geranium, Peppermint, Lemon, Basil

Essential oils for relaxation and stress relief: Lavendar, Jasmine, Roman chamomile, Vanilla

Essential oils for sleep support: Ylang ylang, Vetiver, Lavendar, Jasmine

When making a massage oil or bath oil, you will need to mix your essential oils into a carrier oil. Due to their potency, essential oils should not be used directly on the skin but rather diluted in a carrier oil. Most essential oils will burn and irritate the skin if used directly on the skin without a carrier oil. Good carrier oils are: Jojoba oil, Apricot kernel oil, Almond oil or Grapeseed oil.

Making a massage oil to use topically or in the bath:

Measure out 1/8 cup, 1 oz, or 30 ml of your carrier oil into a glass or ceramic container. To every 1 oz of carrier oil, you can add up to 8 drops of essential oils. Start by adding just 3-4 drops of your essential oils to your carrier oil, shake well, and let it sit for a few minutes. Then test your blend by applying a few drops to the back of your hand. If the scent is too faint, continue adding essential oils one drop at a time until you reach your desired strength. I like to let the essential oils permeate the carrier oil for 2 weeks, shaking the bottle every few days, before I use them.

Making a room spray:

Start with a glass bottle with a spray lid. You want a colored bottle such as brown (amber) or blue tinted glass bottle. The colored bottle will protect the essential oils from oxidative damage thereby helping your spray last longer. Add 1 tsp or 2 ml of non-flavored alcohol (such as vodka) to your clean empty bottle. The alcohol will preserve and fix the essential oils. Add 5-10 drops of essential oils per 1 oz of water. If using a 4 oz bottle, start with adding 20 drops of essential oils then add water to fill the bottle. Shake the bottle vigorously and then do a test spray. Move to a location away from where you have been mixing your oils to get a clean test. Spray into the air or over your head and let the mist fall. If the mist too light in scent, add 5 more drops of essential oils. Keep adding 5 drops until you have reached your preferred strength up to a maximum of 10 drops per 1 oz of water.

Bioidentical Hormone Replacement Therapy

My Ideal Health Model

My theoretical model for perfect health comes from understanding how the body is made and how it functions under the best conditions. If the body was working perfectly and had no stressors on it – no illness, no genetic mutations, no structural misalignments, no environmental, emotional or psychological issues – how would it function? During perimenopause and menopause, how would the body maintain hormone balance and health naturally without modern medicine?

A woman would put on some weight and increase her fat distribution. At the same time her daily physical activity, probably 3-4 hours of physical activity daily, would maintain her muscle strength, agility, bone density and heart health. Her diet would consist of smaller amounts of animal protein from animals that ate plants in their environment (not corn and soy) or fish that were living in clean water which would give her an improved fatty acid ratio. The main part of her diet would be plant based – vegetables and fruit which varied seasonally depending on where she lived with a small amount of whole, unprocessed grains or carbohydrates. Her individual diet would vary based on where she lived and her health challenges would also be affected by her local environment. She would not base her health by what she saw in the mirror or on social media images. She would also die younger than we do today due to accidents and lack of access to medical intervention for infections, but she might also be healthier and more vital up until her death with less diabetes, heart disease, and cancer.

We live in a different world. We want to stay healthy and happy and not gain weight. We have many, many ways we can spend money to enhance our looks and appear younger and we do. The "anti-aging movement" is an incredible money maker in the U.S., Europe, and Asia. We do not spend the majority of our day in movement but rather seated; we eat more calories than would be possible without modern technology, and we have evolved our wants and needs to encompass a much more complex and stimulating life. Our wealth and fortune are both wonderful and problematic. We have much fewer limitations and much greater opportunities to live the life we want and to live longer than the women who came before us.

Our environment has a significant impact on our health, and we cannot separate ourselves from the world we live in. For these reasons, many women will not be able to have the hormone balance they desire with herbal medicine and supplements alone. In years past it was easier to accomplish this. Our environment was cleaner, and we had not yet been drenched in the chemicals now present in every inch of Earth's surface and global water supply. Many by-products of chemicals in our environment impact our hormones and the hormone receptors in our body. When these foreign chemicals enter our bodies through water, food, and the air we breathe, they find our hormone receptors and fit into them like a key fitting into a lock. When these receptor sites are filled, the brain gets the signal that there are plentiful hormones in the body, and it shuts down hormone production. Remember our discussion of the endocrine system? The brain controls production and release of hormones based on the signals it is receiving from the glands and cells.

Most menopausal women I test have lower than optimal hormone levels. They not only have low hormones compared with fertile levels, but they are lower than what they should be during menopause. Why do so many women have low hormones after menopause? I think much of this is a dysfunction in the hormone receptors. We are seeing this in younger women and young men these days as well. There has been an incredible surge in the number of women in their 20's and 30's who have metabolic syndrome or polycystic ovary syndrome. Both conditions involve high levels of the 'male' hormones and a decrease in progesterone and/or estrogen. Residue and breakdown products from chemicals that have been used in agriculture, plastics, manufacturing, landscaping and pest abatement for many decades have found their way into the water supply, food chain, and into the air we breathe. These chemicals disrupt our hormones by attaching to hormone receptor sites and making our body think there is an excess of hormones when there is not. These chemical hormone disruptors are major contributors to infertility, painful periods, lack of periods or irregular periods, acne and PMS.

When Hormones Are Needed

What are bioidentical hormones?

Bioidentical hormones are hormones made in a lab from organic substances that have the same chemical and physical structure as the hormones we make naturally. Unlike bioidentical hormones, synthetic hormones like those found in birth control pills have a completely different biochemical structure than what our bodies make. Both bioidentical and synthetic hormones influence our bodies, but synthetic hormones are not utilized, absorbed, or broken down by the liver in the same way our natural hormones are.

Let's look at other bioidentical hormones that are used in everyday medical practice – thyroid hormones. The medications Synthroid, levothyroxine, Cytomel and liothyronine are all bioidentical thyroid hormones. They have the same chemical structure as the thyroid hormones made naturally by our thyroid glands. All these thyroid medications are made in the lab, but they have the same biochemical structure as our own thyroid hormones. If we do not take artificial thyroid hormones when we have low thyroid hormone production, why would we take artificial estrogen or progesterone if those were low? Comparing thyroid hormone replacement therapy with bioidentical hormone replacement therapy can help people understand why one would consider bioidentical hormone therapy in perimenopause or menopause.

When a woman is experiencing symptoms of low sex hormones and her hormone levels have been tested and she has tried treatments to improve her body's own production of hormones and those treatments have failed, then bioidentical hormone treatment is an option. Our goal should be the same for bioidentical sex hormone therapy as it is for thyroid hormone therapy – bring hormone levels to normal levels for a woman's age and maintain them there. For women in perimenopause we want to allow her hormones to come down to menopausal levels over time just as they would naturally. Eventually they will come down low enough to where she will stop her periods and go into menopause. After menopause we want to keep women's hormones in the normal **menopausal range**, not bring her back up to menstruating levels. We keep a woman in the normal range by monitoring her symptoms and doing regular hormone tests to verify that hormones are indeed in the normal range. This is how we keep women in a safe range and keep her at low risk for hormone related cancers.

Benefits of Bioidentical Hormone Treatment

We live in a time of great research. Since 1997 when I began practicing, the wealth of information and clarity from research on hormones and how they influence health and aging has been dramatic. We know so much more about hormones and their effect on long term health than we ever have. We need to know this. We are living much longer than we were just a few generations ago, and the large baby boomer generation has supported much of the medical research on healthy aging and longevity. We have a wealth of information regarding what people need to live longer with a high quality of health and wellness.

An important finding that has come out of hormone replacement therapy research is the timing of when a woman begins hormone replacement therapy. For women who start low dose hormone replacement therapy within 10 years of menopause there is little to no increased risk for hormone related cancers. But for women who start hormone replacement therapy 10 years or more after menopause, there is a small increased risk. Once a woman has had low hormone levels for 10 years or more, the increase in estrogen from hormone replacement therapy can act as a fuel for hormonally mediated cancer cells that have laid dormant due to hormone deprivation. Once they are fed hormones, these dormant cells can become active and progress into tumor formation.

Research over the last 15 years has shown the benefits of maintaining normal hormone levels in both women after menopause and men after andropause. Low estrogen levels have been shown to increase the risk for both dementia and Alzheimer's in women and low testosterone levels are associated with cognitive decline in men. Estrogen also shows a protective effect on the heart and new research is showing a correlation with normal estrogen levels being associated with improved cholesterol processing. We have long known of the effects of estrogen, progesterone, and testosterone on the bones. Low levels of all hormones show an increase in bone loss and increased risk for osteoporosis. But even more potent in long term health are the effects of chronic sleep disorders and mood disorders and their accumulative effect on aging and disease. Bioidentical hormone replacement therapy can assist many women in improving sleep and mood disorders without medication. For all the aforementioned possible benefits, maintaining hormone balance can be a key player in lifelong health, wellness, and disease prevention.

How do you use bioidentical hormones?

Bioidentical estrogen can be used in a cream form, vaginal insert or suppository or transdermal patch. Bioidentical progesterone can be used in a cream form, vaginal suppository, or oral capsule. For women, testosterone should only be used in a cream form when needed. I do not recommend estrogen in an oral form as higher dosages are needed to make it through the liver and digestive tract. Transdermal application of estrogen (in a cream, patch, or suppository form) does not increase clotting or cause clotting problems since it bypasses liver on first pass. Oral dosing of estrogen has an increased likelihood of causing clotting issues in susceptible individuals.

The best form of bioidentical hormones depends on the woman using them. For example, the transdermal patch is not a good option for women who swim regularly or have frequent and extended water exposure. For women who have difficulty maintaining a regular routine of cream application, the cream form is not optimal. For women with more significant vaginal dryness, a suppository can be more effective at relieving symptoms. For women with difficult to treat sleep problems, oral progesterone may be more effective than the cream form. For these reasons I recommend working closely with your practitioner to get labs done to verify your hormone levels, determine which form of hormones is best for you, and monitor symptoms and labs to maintain hormone balance. During perimenopause, this is a more difficult process. Hormones are in flux and their levels can vary from month to month. Dosing with bioidentical hormones can require more frequent evaluation and adjustment to help a woman progress through perimenopause while keeping her symptoms at manageable levels. After menopause the hormones are much more stable and finding a dose that will work long term is easier.

Research Studies on Hormones and Long-Term Health

The following research studies relate to hormones and their role in specific health conditions as well as in overall longevity. These studies begin to clarify the picture of the role hormones play in preventing disease as we age. There is always more research that needs to be done, but these and other recent studies further our understanding of the use of hormones in maintaining health after menopause.

Hormones and Heart Health

Recent research by Dr. Ferdinand Roelfsema, Rebecca J. Yang, and Dr. Johannes Veldhuis published in the *Journal of the Endocrine Society,* focused on hormone therapy and heart health. This study was unusual in that is looked specifically at bioidentical hormones instead of synthetic hormones which have been used in most of the previous studies on hormones and heart health. The study showed that the group of women who used bioidentical estrogen alone without progesterone had improved cholesterol values. Previous studies have questioned progesterone's effect on the heart, and many practitioners have questioned whether synthetic progesterone has a different impact on heart health than bioidentical progesterone. A second group of women in Roelfsema et al's study used bioidentical progesterone with bioidentical estrogen and showed improvement in cholesterol values except for a mild decrease in HDL, the beneficial cholesterol. This result was better than what had been found previously in women who used synthetic progesterone whose cholesterol values had worsened.

Roelfsema F, Yang RJ, Veldhuis JD. Differential effects of estradiol and progesterone on cardiovascular risk factors in postmenopausal women. *J Endo Soc.* **2018;2(7):794-805.**

I would like to see many more studies on using bioidentical hormones and transdermal hormones versus oral estrogen and synthetic progesterone. The way we apply hormones and the type of hormone we use would logically have different impacts on the way our bodies utilize those hormones.

Another wonderful study was done in Iceland with almost 3,000 women examining the long term use of hormone replacement therapy and its effect on heart disease risk. The researchers used coronary artery calcium scoring, a test done to determine the amount of plaque buildup in the arteries as their marker for heart disease risk. What the researchers found was that women who used hormone replacement therapy had lower plaque buildup overall and the longer they had been on hormones, the lower their plaque buildup was. For women who had been on hormones for fifteen years or more their coronary calcium scores were 50% lower than for the women who had never used hormone replacement therapy. The greatest benefit appeared to be for women who had started hormone replacement therapy within five years of menopause.

Long term hormone replacement is associated with low coronary artery calcium in a cohort of older women: The AGES-Reykjavik Study *Journal American Geriatrics Society* **2017 Jan; 65(1): 200–206.**

In *2017 the American College of Cardiology* at their annual conference presented research on women living longer with less incidence of disease overall when they had used hormone replacement therapy. In addition, they highlighted research being done internationally showing a lower risk for heart disease in women using hormone replacement therapy.

Menopause Societies Revise Stance on Hormone Replacement Therapy

The International Menopause Society and the *North American Menopause Society* have been very cautious about hormone replacement therapy over the last 20 years. They review all the research related to hormones and long term health. In 2016 they came out with a new, bold statement regarding hormone therapy. They noted that hormone therapy was the most effective and safest treatment for menopause symptoms and for issues related to bladder and vaginal tissue health. Both societies focus extensively on lifestyle factors such as smoking cessation, decreasing alcohol use, and maintaining normal weight as cornerstones for long term health. Their recent reversal of their position on hormone therapy from concern and caution to acknowledgment of its long term benefits and safety was very significant. They reference the mounting data on prevention of bone loss, decrease in heart disease, and overall improvement in long term health and wellness in women who begin hormone replacement therapy around menopause.

Preventing Health Issues Associated with Menopause

One of the benefits of practicing for over twenty years is seeing people go through different phases of life. After having worked with thousands and thousands of patients, I have become familiar with the health challenges people face as they get older. Working with women from adolescence through their senior years, I see trends emerge related to conditions that are separate from yet also related to hormone changes. There are the more minor and bothersome issues of hair loss and decreased libidos that upset many women in menopause, but as a doctor, I am even more concerned about the major health issues of sleep disorders, heart disease, cognitive decline and psychiatric issues we can prevent and treat by maintaining hormone balance. If we are able to help a woman return to normal sleep patterns, decrease unaccounted for anxiety or depression, maintain normal blood pressure and heart rhythm and maintain or slow the decline of cognitive function by balancing her hormones then we are also decreasing her need for medications and more risky interventions that have long term side effects. We want to decrease a woman's overall risk for disease while also increasing her longevity and wellbeing throughout her life. The following articles demonstrate the associated issues that women face in menopause that hormone therapy may address.

Questions to Consider Regarding Depression, Sleep Disorders, Heart Disease and Their Treatments

Depression

Kaiser Permanente, one of the few remaining health management organizations, has been a leader in medical research and preventive care. Their research shows that one in five women will experience significant depression in her lifetime. They calculate that fifteen percent of all women will take antidepressants, but for women in the 40 to 59-year-old age group this percentage increases to twenty three percent.

When a woman develops depression around menopause that is not related to situational or life events, it is wise to consider what treatments she has available to her and what the risks of those treatments are. Initial treatments for mood support include dietary changes including a decrease in alcohol use, a supportive exercise routine, social support and activities that support her emotional wellbeing, but if a woman is not able to integrate these changes into her life because of the severity of her depression or if these changes do not yield a significant change in her mood, more intensive treatments need to be considered. Anti-depressant medications can be used, but we must also look at their short and long term safety. Hormone therapy may also be an option in reestablishing normal neurotransmitter production and mood. When determining treatment options, we can assess and compare the risks associated with anti-depressant use with the risks associated with hormone therapy.

Sleep Disorders

The American Heart Association reported that sleep disorders increase the risk for diabetes and obesity while also increasing the risk for heart disease. A great number of women experience sleep issues during perimenopause and into the senior years. Some women use over the counter medications to help with sleep and some will use prescription medications. Other women use herbal formulas and hormone therapy to help with sleep. We are now seeing an increase in women using cannabis products to help with sleep. What we need to consider is the short term and long term effects of the treatments themselves. We know that not treating sleep disorders has health consequences, but what are the consequences of treatments? Some over the counter sleep aids will have a negative impact on kidney and cognitive function with long term use. Prescription sleep medications can have a negative impact on cognitive function and can be habit forming if used for many years. We as of yet have no idea what the impact of long term cannabinoid, THC, or overall cannabis use is as it has not yet been studied in this way. If we can help a woman return to normal sleep cycles with the use of hormone therapy, does her decreased risk for diabetes and heart disease outweigh her risk of taking hormones? These are the complex questions to discuss with your health care provider. Our life expectancy has greatly increased over the last generation so we must now assess the long term impact treatments have on our longevity.

Hormone Therapy and Cancer Risk

The big question almost every woman ponders when deciding whether to use hormones during perimenopause and after menopause is whether this will increase her cancer risk. Cancer has increased exponentially over our lifetimes. Looking at what will contribute to or decrease our cancer risk over our lifetimes is crucial. The data has been conflicting over the last thirty years as to whether hormone therapy contributes significantly to our cancer risk or not. Though we still do not have all the details as to what exactly causes cancer in each woman, we do know much more about what can contribute and by how much.

Some cancers are fed by estrogen and progesterone including ovarian cancer, uterine cancer, and some forms of breast cancer. We know that women who make a high amount of estrogen naturally during their menstrual years are at increased risk for cancer. We also know that women who are estrogen dominant, who have a higher amount of estrogen in relation to their progesterone levels are also at an increased risk for both gynecological problems as well as hormonally mediated cancers. Genetic research is also beginning to elucidate which genetic mutations related to how women process hormones increase cancer risk.

Long term studies in the United States and United Kingdom have come up with some cancer risk assessments regarding hormone therapy. These studies involved large groups of women over many years who were using mostly conventional hormone replacement therapy at patented dosages. They were not using bioidentical hormones in individualized dosages. They did not have their hormone levels tested regularly to determine whether their hormone levels were in normal ranges for their age, and many took their hormones orally instead of transdermally. From these studies they found that estrogen therapy alone without progestins (synthetic progesterone) can cause a small increased risk for ovarian and uterine cancer. When combining estrogen therapy with progestins, there was no increased risk for these cancers. For breast cancer there is a small increased risk for combination estrogen-progestin therapy. It is very interesting to look at the calculated increased risk for these cancers. For the above described increased risks, from the American Cancer Society, for breast cancer "…if 10,000 women took EPT (estrogen-progesterone therapy) for a year, it would result in up to about 8 more cases of breast cancer per year than if they had not taken hormone therapy." For ovarian cancer, "…if 1,000 women who were 50 years old took hormones for menopause for 5 years, one extra ovarian cancer would be expected to develop."

Practitioners like myself question whether this risk would be even lower for low dose individualized bioidentical hormone replacement therapy. In my practice I have seen women on conventional hormone therapy that when I tested their hormone levels, they were estrogen dominant and progesterone deficient. Many had been given hormones for years without ever having their hormone levels checked. For the women I work with I require annual hormone labs to confirm that their hormones are within the normal range for their age. We want to prevent high hormone levels to keep cancer risk low. Further research needs to be done comparing conventional hormone therapy with bioidentical hormone therapy where estrogen is administered transdermally along with bioidentical progesterone, in small individualized doses to women who have their hormone levels checked regularly.

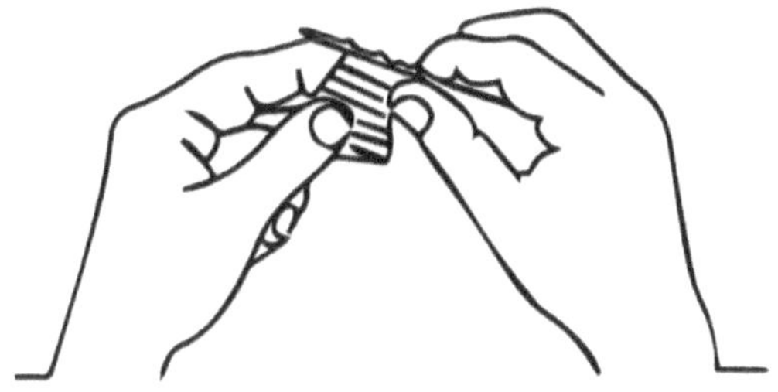

Weaving It All Together

Being a woman is an amazing experience especially when we are able to move from feeling out of control and miserable to feeling re-energized and calm. My hope is that this book clarifies perimenopause and menopause and takes the mystery out of why women feel the way they do when their hormones are out of balance. We can move forward with grace and peace when we realize we can help ourselves feel better and make our hormones work for us instead of against us. As we develop new ways of caring for ourselves, we will feel a renewed sense of happiness and vitality. Our bodies can now be our allies as we move into the next phase of our lives ready to meet new challenges and make new discoveries.

Perimenopause and menopause are long, winding journeys, and they are different for each woman. Honor where you are on the path and the challenges you have already faced. Acknowledge what you have learned and the new skills you are trying out. It is going to be awkward at times as you deal with a changing body with changing needs. You are learning about your new self, and there is much to be discovered. You now have the tools to support your body through these changes and to calm your mind and emotions to be more present in your life.

There might be feelings of loss and sadness that arise as some of what has been falls away, and it can be helpful to give those feelings some time and attention. Just remember that there is also new life being born, and this next part of your life will also be an adventure with opportunities for joy and happiness. As we step away from the fear of the unknown and feelings of loss about what was, we get to embrace the present moment, and the opportunities for future moments. In these present moments we can find happiness again and a new sense of purpose and meaning. Life is still opening up for greater experiences, and we are still becoming!

Practice 10 – Putting it All Together

Let's gather up all that we have discovered to create a map of the journey ahead. You are preparing to birth this next part of your life and yourself. The map you create will help you stay focused, remembering what you are going through and what tools you have at your disposal to deal with what comes up along the way. It will also keep you inspired when the going gets rough.

A Collage of Your Journey - Collages are a visual representation of our conscious and unconscious minds helping us create a literal and figurative map. You are inviting both your conscious self as well as your unconscious creative mind to play here.

Collect images from Pinterest, magazines, old photos, catalogs, brochures or old wall calendars. Sort through images in a relaxed manner, allowing the pictures to speak to you. What images draw your attention, inspire you, or excite you? Do not think about an image but rather let your feelings about it lead the way. You may gather a large pile of images initially and then sort through them again, discarding those that no longer feel right.

Next pick out a background or base for your collage. Choose the medium that most resonates with you for the backbone of your collage. Do you want a two-dimensional collage on poster board or a notebook cover? Or are you visualizing a three-dimensional form on a piece of wood or papier mache? You cannot do in wrong. Let your feelings and creativity lead the way.

With your background in mind, begin to cut out or prepare your images to attach to the background. What details will you keep and which are extraneous? Are you including photos of yourself, your family, your dwelling, your art or profession, where you want to travel, activities you are looking forward to? Or is your collage more abstract with images, textures, colors that speak to you more symbolically? When you are ready, attach your images to your background then stand back and admire!

Your creation may not make immediate sense to you. Sometimes it will take months or even years for the meaning of images to become clearer. This will also be part of your becoming, discovering where your creative mind is leading you.

List of Practices

Practice 1 – Telling Your Story

Give yourself time to do this exercise. It may take a few sittings to fully recollect and reflect to be able to tell your own Secret Life of Hormones story.

Puberty and Your First Period
Think back to puberty. Do you remember when you first heard about girls having their periods? How did you feel when you were anticipating the start of your period? Was it scary? Exciting? Horrifying?

What were those first years of your period like for you? Did you take it in stride, or did it have a big impact on your life? Did your period come every month or was it sporadic?

Did you start before your friends or after your friends? Did you feel different about yourself and about the world once you had started your period?

Fertility and Pregnancy
What are your first memories around being able to get pregnant? Did you cherish the idea of becoming a mother or did the idea having a child make you uncomfortable? Was becoming a mother a major desire for you in your life or did you want to put your time and energy into other endeavors?

How did you feel about getting pregnant? Were you able to get pregnant easily or did you need assistance? Was it stressful? Exciting? Scary? Joyful?

If you had multiple children, what did the process of pregnancy and birthing children mean to you? As you went through this enormous life change of birthing children, how did your thoughts and feelings about yourself change? Did you think of the world differently?

If you were unable to become pregnant but wanted to get pregnant, how did you feel about not being able to get pregnant? How did you feel about yourself and the world when you were not able to become pregnant?

If you did not go through pregnancy and did not want to become pregnant, what was it like seeing friends and family go through pregnancy? Did your feelings about yourself and the world change as you went through this time in your life?

Practice 2 – The Perimenopausal Years

What is your experience with perimenopause: are you experiencing hormonal changes yourself? Have you seen it in your friends, sisters, mother or aunts? What have you learned from other women who are going through this change or have already been through it?

If you are seeing hormonal changes within yourself, describe what is different? Is your period changing or have PMS symptoms changed? Are you experiencing hot flashes, increased irritability, or sleep problems?

As you read over the symptoms associated with estrogen and progesterone and their actions in the body, do you see any patterns with your own symptoms?

If you have been through perimenopause and are now in menopause, think back about what your transition was like. Did you know what you were going through at the time? What was it like going through the body and mind changes? How did you think and feel about yourself as you went through these changes?

For many women this transition takes many years. As you look back, can you see your progression through perimenopause and how you changed during that time? Do you feel differently about your world now that you are in menopause?

Practice 3 – Tracking Symptoms

Start a symptom journal or load a health app onto your phone where you can keep track of symptoms. You do not need to know why you are having symptoms or if any of your discomforts are related to hormonal change. Just keep a list of health issues that bother you on a consistent basis to share with your health practitioner.

If you are still having a period monthly or irregularly, download an app to track your periods. Many apps also help you track other symptoms throughout the month.

Keep notes about changes in sleep, new headaches patterns, herpes outbreaks, yeast infections and mood changes.

Practice 4 – Sex

How is sex going for you? What is your history around sex: has it been more pleasure or pain? How is it changing at this point in your life?

Has your libido changed? Do you dread sex or miss sex?

Are you having any problems with sex?

Have libido changes or problems with sex impacted your relationship with your partner? Does your partner seem to be going through any changes with sex or libido?

Consider whether it would be beneficial to engage in a conversation with your partner around sex. Would making adjustments to your love making make it more pleasurable for each of you?

Practice 5 – The Question of Aging

The topic of aging is a huge one. What came up for you as you read the section on aging? What feelings and thoughts arose? What was uncomfortable or downright frightening?

How have you felt about aging up to this point in your life? Consider what role models you have regarding getting older. Are there some that inspire you? What is it about them that makes you feel good?

If you do not know anyone who is aging in a way that you want to emulate, consider expanding your view. Actively seek out a model of healthy aging - a neighbor, a friend's parent, a coworker, an actor, an athlete, the usher at your local performing arts center. Notice what you respect about them.

Begin to describe how you want to be as you get older. How do you want to feel?

What do you want to be doing? What types of activities sound interesting? What new endeavors could you put time into that you have not had time for yet?

How do you want your body to feel? Will you change your style – hair, makeup, or clothing?

These are questions that will take years to answer fully, but as we begin to consider positive aspects of aging, we change our relationship from one of fear and avoidance to one of acceptance and positivity.

Practice 6 – Making Friends with Your Body

How do you feel about your body? Would you say you are friends with your body, foes, or neutral?

Take this moment to close your eyes, sit quietly and feel what it would feel like to be friends with your body. Stay with it for a few minutes, really feel throughout your whole body and into your heart what it would feel like to be best friends with your body.

In your quiet time, imagine what this new body feels like. What does it look like? How does it move?

If negative thoughts come up during this exercise, let them float away. Let any negative feelings, thoughts, or images fade away during your visualization time. This is precious reprogramming time where you get to connect with what you want. Value it and care for it gently. This is part of creating the next iteration of you.

You can take this exercise a step further by creating a vision board for your new body. Collect images of new clothes you may wear, new hairstyles or makeup you may try, new activities you may engage in as you shift your body into this new place. Let yourself get excited about it. You can even start some of these changes now – get that haircut, try on that new style even before your body gets to your goal. You are investing in yourself and you deserve it!

Practice 7 – Making Exercise Work for You

What forms of movement interest you? What have you always wanted to try? What would you secretly love to be able to do?

(See the list of movement inspirations and examples of exercise routines on page 61-62)

I. What 3 physical activities do you enjoy or could see yourself doing:

1.
2.
3.

II. Go through your weekly calendar or schedule. Find 4 time slots where you could fit in movement. If you are not exercising currently, this can be 20 minutes to start with. If you have been exercising, make it 30-45 minute time slot.

1.
2.
3.
4.

III. Create a colorful calendar or find an app for your phone where you can schedule in movement times, set your alarm, or have notifications sent to remind you.

Put your exercise clothes in the car before you go to work. Carry walking shoes with you or leave them at the office for walks during your lunch or breaks. Exercise on your way to work by riding your bike, walking to the bus, or walking to your carpool pick up point. Turn in your high heels for shoes that could be used for walking during the day. Change up your wardrobe a few days a week to allow for lunchtime walks or walking to meetings instead of driving.

Practice 8 – Nourishment

What diets have you heard about that you are curious to try?

What diets have you tried before that worked well and made you feel good but you did not stick with long term? What made it difficult to stay with that diet?

What do you eat that you know your body does not like?

Choose a food plan that interests you and looks realistic for you. Try that plan for 30 days.

Journal about what feelings come up for you as you try new foods.

Record changes in your symptoms: nasal or sinus congestion, changes in bowel movements, upset stomach, gas, bloating, headaches or mood changes. What symptoms were you having regularly before the new 30-day diet? How are your symptoms changing during the 30 days?

When you reintroduce your old foods back into your diet after the 30 days, do some old symptoms return or worsen that had been gone during the month? Avoid focusing on weight during the first 30 days. Your weight will not change much or at all in those first 30 days.

Practice 9 – Creating Your Own Medicine
Making Your Own Herbal Tea

Herbal teas are both enjoyable to drink as well as beneficial for conditions such as intestinal gas and stomach upset, sleep issues, and anxiety. Try Fennel seed tea with Ginger root or Cardamom seeds for gas or slow digestion. For a calming tea, use Holy Basil leaf (Tulsi), Lemon balm leaf, Milky Oats straw or Lavender flowers. To help with winding down to sleep, a combination of Skullcap flowers, leaves, and stems, Lemonbalm leaf, and Passionflower flowers can be used.

Tea Preparation

When making your own herbal teas, consider which part of the herb or plant you are using. For soft parts such as flowers, leaves, and stems, use 1 Tbsp dried herbs per 1 cup of water. Bring the water to a boil and then take it off the heat. Pour water over herbs in a glass or ceramic container and let steep with a lid on for 15-20 minutes, strain the tea then drink warm or cold. When you are using the hard parts of the plant such as seeds, roots, or bark, use 1 tsp of dried herbs per 1 cup of water. In a glass or ceramic pan, simmer the herbs in the water for 15-20 minutes. Then strain the tea and allow to cool. You can store your tea for a few days in the refrigerator. Limit herbal teas to 3 cups per day.

Herbs in Cooking

Herbs such as Ginger root and Turmeric root can be used in cooking to aid digestion and help calm inflammation. In Ayurvedic medicine Ginger and Turmeric are made into a paste often with coconut oil to retain the medicinal constituents in the herbs. This paste is then used in cooking to impart both flavor and health benefits. Cinnamon can be used for blood sugar control and tastes delicious added to oatmeal, smoothies, and apple dishes. Garlic not only adds its unique flavor to Mediterranean dishes, but it is also one of the best anti-viral agents of all time. Flaxseeds used in smoothies, added to yogurt or cereal, or mixed into salad dressings help with regular bowel movements as well as providing moisture to skin and eyes.

What herbs can you add to your diet to enhance your health? Consider experimenting with Ayurvedic dishes, Mediterranean herbs and spices, or making health booster smoothies to enrich your diet and support wellness.

Aromatherapy

What type of formula would you like to create – an oil for the bath; a blend to use topically on the skin; a mix to use in a diffuser or a spray for your room?

What symptom do you most want to treat – sleep issues, low energy and mood, or stress and anxiety? Try one of these blends below or make a trip to your local health food store and sample the essential oils there; then create your own blend!

Essential oils for energy and mood support: Neroli, Grapefruit, Geranium, Peppermint, Lemon, Basil

Essential oils for relaxation and stress relief: Lavendar, Jasmine, Roman chamomile, Vanilla

Essential oils for sleep support: Ylang ylang, Vetiver, Lavendar, Jasmine

When making a massage oil or bath oil, you will need to mix your essential oils into a carrier oil. Due to their potency, essential oils should not be used directly on the skin but rather diluted in a carrier oil. Most essential oils will burn and irritate the skin if used directly on the skin without a carrier oil. Good carrier oils are: Jojoba oil, Apricot kernel oil, Almond oil or Grapeseed oil.

Making a massage oil to use topically or in the bath:

Measure out 1/8 cup, 1 oz, or 30 ml of your carrier oil into a glass or ceramic container. To every 1 oz of carrier oil, you can add up to 8 drops of essential oils. Start by adding just 3-4 drops of your essential oils to your carrier oil, shake well, and let it sit for a few minutes. Then test your blend by applying a few drops to the back of your hand. If the scent is too faint, continue adding essential oils one drop at a time until you reach your desired strength. I like to let the essential oils permeate the carrier oil for 2 weeks, shaking the bottle every few days, before I use them.

Making a room spray:

Start with a glass bottle with a spray lid. You want a colored bottle such as brown (amber) or blue tinted glass bottle. The colored bottle will protect the essential oils from oxidative damage thereby helping your spray last longer. Add 1 tsp or 2 ml of non-flavored alcohol (such as vodka) to your clean empty bottle. The alcohol will preserve and fix the essential oils. Add 5-10 drops of essential oils per 1 oz of water. If using a 4 oz bottle, start with adding 20 drops of essential oils then add water to fill the bottle. Shake the bottle vigorously and then do a test spray. Move to a location away from where you have been mixing your oils to get a clean test. Spray into the air or over your head and let the mist fall. If the mist too light in scent, add 5 more drops of essential oils. Keep adding 5 drops until you have reached your preferred strength up to a maximum of 10 drops per 1 oz of water.

Practice 10 – Putting it All Together

A Collage of Your Journey - Collages are a visual representation of our conscious and unconscious minds helping us create a literal and figurative map. You are inviting both your conscious self as well as your unconscious creative mind to play here.

Collect images from Pinterest, magazines, old photos, catalogs, brochures or old wall calendars. Sort through images in a relaxed manner, allowing the pictures to speak to you. What images draw your attention, inspire you, or excite you? Do not think about an image, but rather let your feelings about it lead the way. You may gather a large pile of images initially and then sort through them again, discarding those that no longer feel right.

Next pick out a background or base for your collage. Choose the medium that most resonates with you for the backbone of your collage. Do you want a two-dimensional collage on poster board or a notebook cover? Or are you visualizing a three-dimensional form on a piece of wood or papier mache? You cannot do it wrong. Let your feelings and creativity lead the way.

With your background in mind, begin to cut out your images to attach to the background. What details will you keep and which are extraneous? Are you including photos of yourself, your family, your dwelling, your art or profession, where you want to travel, activities you are looking forward to?

Or is your collage more abstract with images, textures, colors that speak to you more symbolically? When you are ready, attach your images to your background then stand back and admire!

Your creation may not make immediate sense to you. Sometimes it will take months or even years for the meaning of images to become clearer. This will also be part of your becoming, discovering where your creative mind is leading you.

Appendix A ~ Antioxidants

The Carotenoid Antioxidants

Beta carotene is an antioxidant you have probably heard of from the carotenoid family. It is a precursor to vitamin A in the body which is necessary for normal functioning of the immune system, lungs, eyes and skin. What we now know is that beta carotene is a relatively minor player compared to other members of the carotenoid family that have a huge impact on our health. Below is a list of the major carotenoids including their food sources and major health benefits.

Astaxanthin - found naturally in red algae and marine animals, it is a red pigment we see in crustacean shells and salmon. Astaxanthin has been promoted for smokers to decrease the oxidation to lungs and blood vessels caused by smoking. It has also been seen to enhance male fertility and looks promising for some forms of cancer.

Lutein – is a very well-studied antioxidant found in high concentrations in spinach, kale, Swiss chard, collard greens, beet and mustard greens, endive, red pepper and okra. Lutein shines in its protection of eye tissue. It can help prevent colon cancer when included in the diet over many years and shows promise for other forms of cancer.

Lycopene - found in high concentration in cooked red tomato products like canned tomatoes, tomato sauce, tomato juice and watermelons. Lycopene has been well studied for its protection of the prostate. Studies have also shown benefits to skin health, reduced risk for skin cancer, and cardiovascular system support.

Zeaxanthin – comes from kale, collard greens, spinach, turnip greens, Swiss chard, mustard and beet greens, corn, and broccoli. Zeaxanthin is a great antioxidant for eye health and works synergistically with lutein.

The next big category of antioxidants are flavonoids, offering oxidative protection to the ears, sinuses, upper respiratory system and hormones. Flavinoids have been very well studied and show great promise for decreasing cancer risk.

The Flavonoid Antioxidants

Quercetin and Rutin are bioflavonoids found in the pith of citrus fruit, kale, tomatoes, broccoli and many other vegetables. These bioflavonoids are beneficial to the upper respiratory system including the sinuses; they strengthen blood vessel walls including those in the kidneys; and many studies have shown them to exert protection against cancer as well as being used in cancer treatment.

The large family of Catechins including Epicatechins and Epigallocatechin gallate (EGCG) found in green tea and chocolate, grape skins and dark-skinned berries among other fruit have widespread health benefits. These include cardiovascular benefits including improved cholesterol ratios; protection to nerve cells including central nerve cells in the brain; anti-bacterial properties in the digestive tract supporting beneficial bacteria balance and promising research on cancer prevention.

Isoflavones also belong to the flavonoid family and include daidzein, genistein, and stilbenoids all of which have hormone like effects in the body. The isoflavones have been well researched for their support in maintaining bone health; cognition and brain health; and cardiovascular health. You may have heard of resveratrol, a very well researched stilbenoid that serves as a very potent antioxidant for the heart. These isoflavones may also be protective against some cancers.

Other big players in the flavonoid family include Caffeic acid from coffee bean; Rosmarinic acid from the herbs rosemary, basil, thyme and peppermint; and Curcumin, the medicinal component of turmeric.

Appendix B ~ Minerals

Minerals – The Minor Players

Potassium is well known for its role in muscle and heart health, but even more importantly, it regulates what enters and leaves every cell in the body. Potassium acts as a gate keeper deciding what nutrients get delivered to the cell and which toxins get removed. Without potassium no cell in the body could function properly. It plays a role in maintaining tissue elasticity (an even more important function after menopause), normal liver function, and regulation of nerve and muscle actions. Potassium is a plentiful mineral found in most vegetables and many fruits including potatoes, apples, bananas, spinach, and broccoli. Peas and beans provide potassium as do many nuts, seeds, and fish.

Sodium is a mineral that has developed a bad reputation. Our main source of sodium is salt, and salt makes food taste good so it has been used in excess, especially in processed food. Salt overwhelms our taste buds and becomes the dominant flavor we taste. It is a good trick to cover up tasteless food with the taste of salt. We no longer taste the food itself but rather the salt flavor dominates and makes us want to eat more. Sodium did not start out as a bad mineral, but it has become a problem due to its overconsumption. Excess sodium causes water retention, increased blood pressure and stress on the kidneys. We need to balance our sodium intake with our potassium intake and limit excess salt to help the cells function at top capacity.

Sodium and potassium are buddies in their roles of cell guardians. Sodium, just like potassium, regulates exchange of products in and out of cells and helps maintain water and fluid balance in the body. Sodium is also an essential component of our digestive juices, and without sodium our blood pressure would be too low.

There is an easy trick to balancing sodium and potassium through our diets. By including potassium rich foods, mainly vegetables and fruit we can provide enough potassium to balance sodium as long as we do not overdue the sodium by eating too many processed foods. Include five servings of vegetables and fruit into your daily diet and cook your own foods without the added salt, and you will achieve good potassium/sodium balance.

Iron is needed for our red blood cells in their role of distributing oxygen throughout the body for normal cell and organ system function. Our whole bodies from our brains to our muscles are dependent on oxygen for normal functioning. We are also now understanding iron's role in a healthy immune system and tissue repair, systems we rely upon even more after menopause. Throughout our lives the main way we lose iron is from bleeding during our periods. When the periods stop in menopause, our iron stores should remain normal without having to supplement extra iron.

Red meat is the most potent source of iron in our diets, but iron can also be found in dark green vegetables, legumes, dried fruits, mushrooms and black strap molasses.

Iodine is found mainly in the thyroid gland and in smaller amounts in the breasts. It is necessary to produce thyroid hormones. Food sources include seaweeds, ocean fish, nuts and seeds, raisins, green leafy vegetables.

About the Author

Dr. Zoe (Wells) Zawalick is an integrative medicine doctor practicing in California since 1997. She is a licensed naturopathic doctor with training in Obstetrics, Gynecology, Endocrinology and a degree in Psychology. Her early practice focused on family practice issues and now she specializes in endocrinology and health issues of adults and seniors.

Dr. Zoe maintains a full time practice while also writing books, articles, posts and blogs on women's health issues as well as preventing and treating the health issues women and men face as they age. Her first book is entitled Women's Transformationl Journey.

She has also developed a line of essential oil blends, AromaWellness Blends and herbal medicine tinctures.

Website: www.drzoe.com

Dr. Zoe is in the process of developing webinars and seminars for women interested in learning more about perimenopause and menopause. Please contact her through her website for more information or to share ideas or insight!